M000211760

This book is dedicated to the night my parents had sex and conceived me. If they hadn't done that, I wouldn't exist.

YOU ARE NOT BROKEN

Stop *"Should-ing" All Over Your Sex Life*

KJ CASPERSON, MD

The information presented herein represents the views of the author as of the date of publication. This book is presented for informational purposes only. Due to the rate at which conditions change, the author reserves the right to alter and update their opinions based on new conditions. While every attempt has been made to verify the information in this book, neither the author nor their affiliates/partners assume any responsibility for errors, inaccuracies, or omissions.

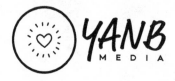

Copyright © 2022 Kelly Casperson
All rights reserved. Reprinting or reusing any or all parts of this book is permitted and encouraged, but only with the written consent of the author.

YOU ARE NOT BROKEN
Stop "Should-ing" All Over Your Sex Life

ISBN HARDCOVER: 978-1-5445-2435-1
      PAPERBACK: 978-1-5445-2434-4
      EBOOK: 978-1-5445-2433-7
      AUDIOBOOK: 978-1-5445-3181-6

CONTENTS

INTRODUCTION 7

PART ONE: It's Not Your Fault! 19

CHAPTER ONE: Society Got It Wrong 21

CHAPTER TWO: "The Rules" Are Ridiculous 35

CHAPTER THREE: Bad Sex Sucks 45

PART TWO: Sex-Positive Sex Ed for Adults 55

CHAPTER FOUR: The Female Edition 57

CHAPTER FIVE: The Male Edition 75

CHAPTER SIX: Getting All Hormonal 85

CHAPTER SEVEN: The Chemistry of Pleasure 95

CHAPTER EIGHT: Own Your Orgasm 99

CHAPTER NINE: Communication Is Lubrication 109

PART THREE: Is It *Actually* Low Desire—or Something Else Entirely? 117

CHAPTER TEN: It Might Not Even Be a "You" Problem 119

CHAPTER ELEVEN: Desire Is SO Two-Faced 129

CHAPTER TWELVE: Brakes and Accelerators   135

CHAPTER THIRTEEN: Get Out of Your Head and Into
Your Body   141

CHAPTER FOURTEEN: Change Your Mind, Change Your Life   151

CHAPTER FIFTEEN: What a Pretty Pink Pill Can (and Can't) Do
for You   157

CHAPTER SIXTEEN: Maybe It's Menopause   175

CONCLUSION: You Are Not Broken   189

ACKNOWLEDGMENTS   193

RESOURCES   195

CITATIONS   199

Introduction

A BOX OF KLEENEX was the only thing I had to offer my sobbing patient who was experiencing low—okay, let's face it, no—sexual desire. It wasn't like a lack of sex was going to end her long-term, loving relationship, but she still felt a huge sense of loss not having that connection with her husband anymore. And even though I was the urologist who'd cured her bladder cancer, I found I wasn't equipped to help her at all with this much-less-life-threatening problem.

As I handed her the tissues, I thought, *I've been to med school. I've spent the past ten years operating in the pelvis. I've looked at more vulvas than 99.9 percent of the people in the world. So why don't I know what to do?* (And by the way, I'm also married with kids and have my fair share of sex. Still nothing.)

Thinking back to when I was a urologist in training, I realized there had been plenty of lectures about the penis but none about the female homologous structures. While I learned everything there is to know about male sexual function, it was like the clitoris—the female equivalent of the penis—didn't even exist. The rare times women's sexual issues actually made it into the conversation, the "experts," who were all males, seemed to write women off as complex and mysterious. It was like, *Don't ask too many questions, we're the professionals here, this is too complicated to be understood—and besides, we don't know anything either.*

Clearly, I was going to have to educate myself for this patient as well as any others who might come to me looking for advice in the future. Furthermore, I was just curious. Why DIDN'T I know this stuff? Did anyone know this stuff? And could MY sex life get better as a result of this knowledge?

I also had an inkling there might be a lot more unspoken and unanswered questions women had about sexual health (though I had no idea at the time just how many there would be). I went on a quest to find out everything I could about women's sexuality. I started telling anyone who would listen what I'd learned.

Since then—in my private urology practice, popular podcast, and weekly (sometimes daily!) Instagram Live Q and A sessions—I've met a lot of other women who, like the crying patient I felt helpless to help, think they're broken because they don't desire or enjoy sex as much as they think they "should." Who are saying yes when a lot of the time what they really mean is no, and then wondering why they're not having desire or fun. Who aren't confident in themselves, can't communicate about their sexual needs, and don't even know how the female sexual body works.

So let's kick things off with a bang—pun intended—by clearing up that misconception: YOU ARE NOT BROKEN. Not only that, but it's time to stop "should-ing" all over your sex life. Thinking you're the problem is a huge burden to put on yourself, and I want to take that weight off you right now. Lack of desire or not enjoying sex "enough" isn't your fault and it's all fixable. I'm going to tell you everything you need to know to have a more satisfying sex life starting today. Seriously. Step one you already know—stop it with all the "shoulds." Self-abuse with shame and guilt is not sexy.

My mission is to help women understand how everything we've learned about sex is wrong. Most of us didn't get a sex education, we got a "disease and reproduction prevention plan." While knowing how to protect yourself from diseases and avoid getting pregnant when you don't want to is valuable, it doesn't have anything to do with female desire, arousal, pleasure, and orgasm.

I want to show you how our bodies and brains really work, in addition to how society uses our sexuality against us, so you can start having great sex again (or maybe even for the first time in your life). This book is for anyone partnered or not, cis-hetero or not—but being partnered in a heterosexual relationship actually has its own specific challenges for women, which we will discuss thoroughly here.

Just the Facts!

Since med school failed to teach me—along with all the other doctors out there—about female sexual function, I made an appointment with Dr. Google. She led me directly to the International Society for the Study of Women's Sexual Health (ISSWSH), which was actually started twenty years ago by a urologist, Dr. Irwin Goldstein. Yay, urology! Who knew? (Dr. Google, apparently.) I started attending meetings, taking advantage of their educational opportunities, and connecting with other people who care about women's sexual health—doctors, nurse practitioners, sex therapists, psychiatrists, and physical therapists. We'd all found our way there because we wanted to help our patients who seemed to have nowhere else to turn.

At the same time, I started reading everything I could get my hands on about the subject. Most of the books I found were either:

1. *call your vagina a yoni; breathe into your spleen (I didn't make this up; it actually said that in a sex help book I read); celebrate your princess goddess warrior.* Lawd. Many of us don't have a religious practice, time to meditate for a half an hour a day, or want to study tantric breathing. Yes,

mindfulness is an amazing way to cultivate pleasure in your life and we will cover it here, but if it's just another "should" on your to-do list, forget about it. Besides, if we all had eight hours a day to spend on our yoni, I'm pretty sure we wouldn't be feeling like we didn't have the time, energy, or desire for sex. Or

2. academic design, small font, written to impress colleagues, and using language and a format so dense you need a PhD to understand or care about it. I have found some seriously dry books about sex, which I previously didn't even know was possible. These books aren't interesting to the average human. Too stuffy and unapproachable.

A small percentage of the books were amazing, though, like *Becoming Cliterate* by Dr. Laurie Mintz, *Come as You Are* by Emily Nagoski, and *She Comes First* by Ian Kerner. This last one, written for men, is chock-full of great information, short sentences, and declarative facts. I thought to myself, *Women need a book like this—Female Pleasure 101, not How to Have Seventeen Different Types of Orgasm with Your Candle-Scented Yoni.*

I capped off my journey by becoming a life coach. I know; I still groan at this name too. How the heck did a surgeon sign up for this woo-woo? Because it is basically ancient philosophy harnessed to help us see our thoughts and challenge them. I was a neuroscience major in college, so I love the brain, and as a urologist, I am already intimately acquainted with female anatomy. Life coaching brings together awareness of our own thoughts, the psychology of the mind, and the physicality of the body parts. I get to use all the best wisdom available to empower women to have the best sex lives possible.

And so here we are. I wrote the book I believe needs to exist for women like you and me, who just want the facts about sex without a heaping serving of unobtainable cosmic bliss on the side. It is the book I wish I had as a younger woman, and that my daughters will now have to refer to when they are old enough to read it.

Who's the Real Authority Here, Anyway?

Are you thinking to yourself, *Hey, maybe that patient of yours just didn't ask the right KIND of doctor for help with her sex drive*? I hear you, but no. Most people assume ob-gyns would be the go-to specialty—I know I did—but they're often too busy helping women have babies and dealing with birth control, unruly periods, STDs, and menopause to take on something as unlifesaving as low libido.

The fact is, there is no "right" doctor to see for female sexual concerns. I ran into an old medical school friend who is a practicing ob-gyn physician at an ISSWSH conference. When I asked, "Why are YOU here?" she told me gynecologists don't get any training on women's sexual health either. Mic drop. Who is taking care of the people sleeping with the people I—as a urologist—am giving Viagra to?

No medical specialty owns this space. It's not surprising when you consider Western medicine is quite patriarchal and focuses on acute illnesses, not chronic "lifestyle" concerns or preventative medicine. Everything was conceived from the male perspective and this is what gets passed down.

Not fun fact: Elizabeth Blackwell, the first woman admitted to an American medical school, was basically let in as a dare. "The faculty, assuming that the all-male student body would never agree to a woman joining their ranks, allowed them to vote on her admission. As a joke, they voted 'yes,' and she gained admittance, despite the reluctance of most students and faculty."[1]

Our medical system was created for and by men. Case in point: until recently, clinical trials for most medications on the market were tested on males only. Since women are not just small men, this is a big problem. Ignoring half of the population leads to limited focus on women-specific issues like pregnancy, menopause, pelvic pain, and female sexual function. Medical school curriculum also barely skims over sex ed. During my entire course of study, only a single classroom session was devoted to sexuality. I remember a video of elderly people having intercourse that the class giggled through. I think the point was that everybody can be sexual despite age or disability—great message—but no one ever explained that to us or delved further into the subject. Watching septuagenarians roll around once was the full extent of our sex-positive education as I remember it.

When I was a medical student interviewing for urology, I was told to do a fellowship (additional training after residency) to specialize in a niche like cancer or kidney stones so I didn't "have to see women." It is just assumed that women are difficult, challenging, and take up too much time. Despite that offensive line of thinking, urologists in general have the funniest and best personalities of all medical specialties, which made it very appealing to me. (In case you're wondering: no, I never did that fellowship. I was never repulsed by women or their pelvis or their "issues." So here I am.)

The Education Gap

So of course I had no idea what to tell the woman crying in my clinic! Like most people, no one ever taught me about female desire, arousal, or pleasure—not my parents, high school sex ed teachers, or even medical school professors—let alone how to stoke it or recover lost desire. I had to learn the way we all do, through sexual partners, equally misinformed friends, unrealistic Hollywood movies, and trial and error. That's not exactly a recipe for great sex.

As of October 1, 2020, thirty states and the District of Columbia require public schools to teach sex education,[2] only twenty-two of which are required by law for that instruction to be medically accurate. A mere eight states and the District of Columbia are mandated to teach about consent, and this is mostly all new since 2019.[3] (This might be why many women feel like they have a difficult time saying no to sex, or end up having it because someone else wants to.)

Let's pick on Texas just for a second: 58 percent of schools there teach abstinence only, and 25 percent don't teach sex ed at all.[4] How do they expect people to have a healthy sex life with such a lack of education?

Even when sex ed is taught, it is so fear-based—it's all about avoiding pregnancy and STIs. No one ever talks about how sex is SUPPOSED to feel great and be fun, or heaven forbid, how to actually bring about that kind of enjoyment, or that normal couples with great relationships can still be flummoxed and devastated by sexual issues. When I tried to find out how many states teach about pleasure, I couldn't find any. Through Planned Parenthood, I finally learned ZERO states are required to include pleasure in their education, which means no one is teaching it at all. No wonder we're so messed up about what we're supposed to be doing and feeling in bed.

I'm thrilled to say that I'm now helping close this sexual education gap. But here's the thing: as a surgeon, I have only fifteen to thirty minutes with a woman in my office. That isn't a great amount of time to break down the three to six decades of bad education, body issues, orgasmic inequality, mountains of shame, nonconsensual sex, and so many "shoulds." Unfortunately, due to the way our medical system works, my clinic isn't the best place for your education.

Get In On the Conversation

All this combined is probably why the whole time I was becoming a "sexpert," there was a voice in my head telling me, *You need to find a way to reach more people than you see in clinic—women NEED to know and hear this.* I tried ignoring that voice for six months but she finally got so annoying, I bought a microphone attachment for my cell phone, went into my closet (I'd read somewhere clothing is good for acoustics), and started my podcast *You Are Not Broken*. An exciting ascent up the Apple charts later, I discovered my deep dive into sexual medicine was both timely and necessary: women have SO MANY unanswered questions about sex, desire, orgasm, menopause, and more. My podcast—and this book—are your safe, comfortable place to learn how to undo the patterns of blame, shoulds, and social conditioning and learn to love the sexual body you have. Yes, woman, you were born to be sexual and enjoy it!

#lifecoach advice: always listen to that little voice inside your head. They say she is your future self, calling you forward. Mine wanted me to be a leader in the women's sexual health revolution. Where will yours take you? What are you going to do with this one great life?

Now that I'm a sexual medicine expert, I just can't keep what I've learned to myself. It's too important for women to know what they're experiencing is common and normal. And even beyond that, it doesn't take a lot of work or money to start desiring and enjoying sex more.

What's most profound to me is that none of what I'm about to tell you is new. It's not like *we just found out vaginal penetration alone doesn't do it for most women but luckily we recently discovered the clitoris!* Plenty of research and books on the topic exist, but the information doesn't seem to be reaching people. And since no one's getting it and everybody needs it, here I am. I hope to create what all the "woo-woo yoni" and dry, boring academic texts haven't yet.

Just to be clear: this book isn't designed as the be-all, end-all of sex education. People teach this in different ways, and I know not everyone will agree with me. Use what's here as a springboard and keep learning. Your sexuality is like a fingerprint—unique among billions—so you will need to do a lot of self-discovery, too. I can't tell you what exactly will work for you. That's for you to find out!

This book also isn't meant to be personal medical advice. I'm a doctor, but in most cases I'm not *your* doctor. The contents here are for informational and entertainment purposes only, and are not intended to diagnose any medical condition, replace the advice of a healthcare professional, or recommend any treatment. Bring your newfound knowledge to your physician team or therapist and work together so you can become as happy and healthy as possible.

My hope is simply that this book starts a conversation—with yourself, your partner, your doctor, or your therapist. That it helps you understand why you think you are broken, and to realize you aren't. That it gives insight into why you're not satisfied, what you can do about it, and how to communicate what you need instead. That it empowers you to see and do things differently from now on, and not just in terms of sex, but in all aspects of your life.

So if you're ready for a wild ride—one that leads to more fun and fulfillment in bed and beyond—read on to learn how:

- society and the media get sex all wrong.
- the female body works, and how it is the same yet differs from male bodies.
- your body has a clitoris that is completely capable of enjoying pleasure—and you carry it around with you twenty-four hours a day (and no, there does not need to be someone naked next to you to use it).
- our limited definition of sex makes it all about male pleasure, and how to expand that definition to include female pleasure.
- a good sex life is up to you—YOU have all the power (no, really!).
- to communicate your needs and desires with your partner, and listen to them in return.

- desire is not one thing, doesn't often come before good sex, and may not be necessary at all (gasp!).

Forget about RE-claiming your sex drive. This is about claiming it possibly for the first time ever. Even better, in most cases, the answers are not outside of you in a pill, toy, technique, or potion— they've always been right there with you (just like your clitoris!).

Borrowing from Glinda the Good Witch here: "You always had the power, my dear, you just had to learn it for yourself." In fact, you will find no one is the expert in your sex life except you. Now you get to start to love and listen and celebrate the "sexpert of yourself" that you always were. Own your authority over your sexuality. It is no one else's to own.

What tone do I want to take in this book? Dry, boring neuroscience data expert? That turns some people off and it has already been done. Sarcastic, snarky, funny sister? Good for some, not others. Ardent feminist? Yes, but not in the "hater of men or society in general" kind of way.

As a lifelong people pleaser, I guess I just have to deal with the fact that not everyone is going to like this book. It will feel "too much" of this and "not enough" of that for some. If that's you, don't worry. I am already thinking those thoughts, so it won't hurt me. If some of this doesn't land well, my sincerest apologies up front. I cannot write a book about sex that will please everyone, but do know I did my best to be accurate and educate the way I would have wanted to be educated (and the way I educated myself), and I'm sorry for any insults or omissions. At the end of the day, I just want to help women and the partners who love them, and make my young daughters proud that their mom tried to make a difference.

I understand this book may sound heteronormative in the sense that I am often talking to (but not assuming) cisgender, vulva-owning, socialized-as-female women. I actually believe cis-hetero women are ignored and sexual minorities, too. Every time I tell people this is my niche, they respond with, "But what about the men, the teenagers, the other humans?" All this tells me is they want to turn my attention off of my target audience, again confirming the bias that women in general don't matter.

I want you to know I believe we should love whomever we want and be gendered however we feel. My worldview is that all are welcome here even though this book focuses on people who have been socialized as women and sleep with humans who have penises (for the sake of this book we'll call them men, although I know that's not always exactly accurate). However, I think everyone will learn something in this book.

One last thing: sex has been used against women since the dawn of time. I hold it very sacred that we all come here with a unique past, and often that includes trauma and abuse. I believe sex and pleasure are innate in everyone and we all have a right to enjoy our bodies. It is what we were given to experience Earth, the power for this lies within us, and no one can take that away without our permission. People can heal and take back their power. Trauma-informed therapy or coaching is an important part of many people's journey to thriving and I strongly encourage this. Sometimes you can't do it alone. Oh, and if I really thought I could write a book that wouldn't offend anyone, either:

1. I shouldn't let anyone read it; or
2. It shouldn't be about sex.

This book is my advocacy work. When a person's passion combines with helping others it is called their dharma. This is mine. Enjoy!

PART ONE

It's Not Your Fault!

CHAPTER ONE

Society Got It Wrong

WHY DO WOMEN find themselves so confused and ambivalent about sex? I blame the mixed messages sent by society, religious traditions, the media, and other institutions that both want our attention and to control us. I see that power play played out in many ways every day.

We live in a patriarchal society—defined as a social system in which men hold primary power and are the dominant force in leadership, moral authority, and social privilege—where a woman's value is in her desirability and a man's is in his ability to desire. Men are supposed to be sexual and women are supposed to be desired. They get to be active while we're expected to be passive.

> Desire is both a noun and a verb. As a noun, it means an impulse toward something that promises enjoyment or satisfaction in its attainment. As a verb, it means to strongly wish for or want something.

That is heavy. And it just gets worse.

Society also tells us we should be sexy while passively waiting to attract Prince Charming—but that once he finally gets here, we can't ACTUALLY want to have sex with him, because then we're considered slutty and loose. Well, that is until we marry him, at which time we should want to have sex with him ALL THE TIME. And if we don't, then we are frigid and broken.

Why would our culture tell us men should desire women because of our sexual desirability, and then not allow us to be sexual without shaming us? Why does our value change depending on that availability instead of being based on our intrinsic value as a person and a partner? I'd like to see a world where we're valued for who we are as a human being AND be able to express our own sexual agency.

Sadly, there's more. We're not supposed to desire ANYTHING of our own. We shouldn't desire beauty, because then we're vain. We shouldn't desire having a job and kids, because we couldn't possibly do both well. We shouldn't shoot for the C-suite, because no man wants to marry someone more successful than he is. We shouldn't excel at sports, because then we're too competitive. We aren't ALLOWED to desire anything, then we feel broken because we don't desire anything. It's a trap.

When was the last time you were curious about something? We kind of forget this as an adult. Kids are curious. They explore, then they fall down and get back up. They don't beat themselves up over failing and trying again. Get curious about more desire in your life. What is it you actually want in this one amazing shot at being human? You deserve to desire!

When I ask women in my clinic what they actually want, I am often met with a curious, blank stare. They don't even know at this point. That's not surprising given the confusing, conflicting messages women get from society about women owning their desires.

We're taught to believe our desires make us UN-desirable, and that it's selfish to want anything for ourselves. So we tamp down our dreams and start to accept that it's okay to not have any desires at all. To cap it all off, we think we're broken because we don't desire the ONE thing we're told we're supposed to desire (which, remember, is hot, lusty passion every day once we are married in one style of defined penetrative sex, for all of our lives).

I know. It's f-ed up. Don't get me wrong, I am very thankful for the gifts and privileges I have been given—but to not desire more because I should just be happy with what I've been given is a passive, disempowering way for anyone to live.

Women have to deal with both slut-shaming and prude-shaming. Even our language is stacked against us. A man who sleeps with a lot of people is called "man-whore," but there's no such thing as a "woman-whore"—implying the word is inherently for women. I'm often referred to as a female doctor, but guys aren't called male doctors. So men get to be the default doctor and women get to be the default whore? Raw deal.

It comes as no surprise that the "fake news" we are fed about sex comes from the male perspective. What I mean by that is men are still making most of the movies, news, shows, and content, which means the narrative is written by people who don't know the facts about women, and who tell the story from their perspective—what gets them off and what they desire. Reese Witherspoon recently commented that Hollywood is outdated in its repetitive, narrow stereotypes, and I agree with her.[5] These stereotypes aren't our reality, but we accept them just the same.

Think any of this is new? Nope. Aristotle once wrote that women are defective by nature. "A female is an incomplete male, or as it were, a deformity."[6] We've endured inferior treatment since the Greek and the Roman times, and probably even before then. It's time for a cultural upgrade! It is time for a female narrative.

This is how society tries—and often succeeds—to control our sexuality, and I'm here to point that out because we don't often see the water we swim in. It's time to take back our power. You have every right to want more than you feel you've been given permission to. It's time to lay claim to your sexual life.

Undoing the Damage

We can start by throwing pretty much all of what we learned about sex out the window. Everything society taught us is wrong. Wow, that's a big claim...*everything* is wrong? Well, at least close to it. Okay, maybe not the "sperm reaches egg and baby is made" part. But the rest of it, yes.

Case in point: society tells us that a penis in the vagina equals sex and everything else ISN'T sex (from now on, I'll call it PIV sex, and no, I didn't invent the term). Remember when President Bill Clinton denied having sex with his intern? This incredibly narrow definition of sex is what allowed him to make such a preposterous claim.

PIV sex focuses on the male pleasure experience. While men tend to orgasm three to five minutes after vaginal penetration—OMG yes, people do actually research and time this stuff—women only EVER orgasm 20 to 30 percent of the time with PIV sex, and certainly not in under five minutes. This doesn't mean we're broken.

It means we're women, living in women's bodies, needing a different kind of arousal and sexual experience.

We have different hardware that actually works very similarly to men's. Unfortunately, we aren't taught to prioritize and stimulate it during our sexual activity. And if we aren't taught this, obviously the penis owners missed the memo too.

So let's start with the basics: the clitoris is our organ of pleasure. Women orgasm with the clitoris, not the vagina. When orgasms actually DO happen during PIV sex, it's because the clitoris has been stimulated THROUGH the vagina (more on this later). PIV sex without added clitoral stimulation is sex that prioritizes male pleasure and leaves women with less pleasure. (Now, not to jump ahead to Advanced Orgasm Graduate School, but some women have been able to orgasm by just thinking their way there, or by stroking a nipple, earlobe, or other body part of choice—but that, number one, is beyond the scope of this book, and two, only goes to prove that the brain is VERY important when it comes to sex.)

Are the psych majors among us thinking about Freud right now, and how he said vaginal orgasms were "mature" and clitoral orgasms were "infantile"? The fact is, the only women having "vaginal orgasms" are having them because of clitoral stimulation. Yet women back then actually had surgeries to move their clitorises closer to their vaginas because Freud said they were deficient for not orgasming with vaginal penetration. Not only was that painful and unnecessary, but it was downright dangerous because there were no antibiotics to treat the inevitable resulting infections. No one—especially Freud—should lie to women and men by telling them their bodies should work in ways they don't.

While we're on the topic of female orgasm...unlike the speedier male experience of three to five minutes after vaginal penetration, it takes women anywhere from thirteen to fifty minutes (depending on the study) to orgasm during partnered sex. Those orgasms happen far more consistently through oral sex, hands, and toys than PIV sex. Why? Because all those tongues, hands, and toys are focusing on the clitoris.

A recent study focused on how long it took women to orgasm after already being "intensely aroused," defined as an "intense desire for sex in presence of erotic stimuli." Results showed the average timeframe then was 13.4 minutes, +/- 7.67 minutes. In that research, 68 percent of women said intercourse alone was insufficient to reach orgasm.[7]

In case you're wondering: yes, women orgasm much faster when doing it alone. Sex researcher Alfred Kinsey discovered it takes women about four minutes to orgasm through masturbation. I personally know women who can do it in less than a minute. Why is that? Because women know what works for them when they are alone.

It is a myth that women take longer. It is a truth that women take longer when their pleasure isn't prioritized (usually in a heterosexual scenario). Side note: rushing to orgasm isn't the goal in general, in case you missed that point. It's not a race. Allow your partner to spend the appropriate amount of time focusing on your pleasure and you'll be amazed by the results.

If you hate the term masturbation—maybe you were taught it's wrong (for many reasons, one being that women are supposed to "save" their sexuality for their partner), or if you touched yourself you'd end up in hell or just be a "bad girl"—perhaps you'll prefer this term for it: self-cultivation. Sounds fancy, right? (I got it from one of those "woo-woo" books.) Like you're getting to know your body and mind—which you are. Like you are indulging in some well-earned self-care. If that's the case, don't

masturbate, self-cultivate! Also, self-cultivating is something you do alone. Nobody's watching you or judging you.
No one needs to give you permission to self-cultivate. It
is natural and healthy (many studies have been done on
this). But if you need permission from a doctor—got you!
Permission granted.

In his 1953 report, *Sexual Behavior in the Human Female,* Kinsey wrote, "There is widespread opinion that the female is slower
than the male in her sexual responses, but the masturbatory data
do not support that opinion. The average male may take something
between two and three minutes to reach orgasm unless he delib-
erately prolongs his activity, and a calculation of the median time
required would probably show that he responds not more than
some seconds faster than the average female. It is true that the average female responds more slowly than the average male in coitus,
but this seems to be due to the ineffectiveness of the usual coital
techniques." Shere Hite echoed his conclusion in her groundbreak-
ing 1976 book, *The Hite Report.* "It is, obviously, only during inad-
equate or secondary, insufficient stimulation like intercourse that
we take 'longer' and need prolonged 'foreplay.'...Women don't need
'foreplay' in masturbation to orgasm."

See what I told you about none of this being new information?
Kinsey was telling people way back in 1953 that PIV sex doesn't do
it for most women. Hite came along and reiterated that in 1976. And
both agreed that the "fact" that women take longer to orgasm than
men is actually just more fake news. We only take longer in heterosexual relationships that prioritize PIV sex over all other methods,
and his orgasm over hers. Otherwise, NO, we are not inherently less
arousable or more difficult to please, so stop "shoulding" on yourself
for not having orgasmic pleasure fast or at all with PIV sex.

On my Instagram Lives, women often ask me, "Why can't women just have orgasms faster during sex?" The answer is, because we don't have penises we're putting in vaginas. If you're in the mood for a quickie, self-cultivate, teach your guy what works for you (after you have figured it out yourself by trial and error and compassionate curiosity), or bring toys into the bedroom to help you both along.

Also, why is this a goddamn race? Oh America, land of the five-minute home loan. Sigh. It's in our blood. Why are we trying to rush this experience like a "to-do" list? What's wrong with taking more time? What's wrong with more pleasure? Orgasms are easier when we are enjoying the process. When time management is the goal instead of pleasure, don't wonder where your orgasm went.

And as for the follow-up question, "Well then, why aren't we built to have orgasms with penises in our vagina?" One theory about why our pleasure bits are on the outside is that the woman needs to feel good and willing to put something in the vagina, which is what allows us to reproduce. Basically, we evolved to get our pleasure first. Modern people seem to have forgotten this fact and rush into what we have been taught "sex" is too quickly.

In another recent study, participants were asked to focus on the woman and her pleasure for at least twenty minutes. Here the rate of female orgasm goes up to 90 percent. Women's bodies need a little bit more time in partnered hetero sex, and do just great given that time. So why do we keep striving for a graduate degree in penis-in-the-vagina sex? A PhD in PIV? Ha!

Yeah, I know. Hopefully you are feeling loved and feeling seen and we have just gotten started.

If you are upset or bothered by not having an orgasm through vaginal penetration, it does not mean that you have sexual dysfunction. It means you didn't get an education that kindly told you that the clitoris is why women orgasm, and sometimes the clitoris is activated through the vagina, but that isn't the only or "gold standard" way. You also didn't get told that about 70 percent of women don't orgasm through vaginal penetration alone. So, you don't need a pill, and you should immediately stop taking on the burden of feeling crappy about yourself when, in fact, it is society that did a crappy job of 1) not teaching you in the first place and 2) allowing you to feel like you need to be fixed. You can still have an orgasm with PIV sex, but make sure to play with the clitoris and the tissue under the labia majora (which is also part of the clitoris) first. Get your erectile tissue involved. Experiment to find out what positions work better than others and get hands, mouth, lube, and/or vibrators involved.

You're More than Enough—and Never Too Much

In society, women are constantly bombarded with people telling us we're not enough. That can have a devastating effect on our confidence and self-worth, especially when it comes to sex. For example, I recently had a patient come to see me at my urology clinic. Before I started my exam, she apologized profusely. She said, "Just so you know, it's really ugly down there. I'm so sorry you have to look at it."

I told her, "I look at labias every day. I've probably seen thousands at this point. I'll be happy to let you know where you land on my 'labial bell curve.'"

I did the exam and found her labia to be very average. Boring. Middle of the road. Happily forgettable. There was nothing abnormal there. There wasn't even anything interesting about it.

I told her, "You're wonderfully average. Top of the bell curve for you!"

Her husband said, "See, I told you! It's absolutely fine."

My patient was blown away. In happy tears, she explained that her ex-husband told her it was ugly at the beginning of their relationship and she'd been hanging onto that thought ever since. How sad to realize she'd limited her pleasure and sexuality for decades over a mean comment (and by a non-vulvar expert), who, if he did have a bell curve of his own, was likely limited to a few individuals or media with "production-quality labias" on it).

Screw that ex-husband and his judgment. My patient and her labia were PERFECT—as in, perfectly normal.

And what about the opposite: when society tells us we're TOO MUCH? A sexually confident woman is equally challenged by the rules. Think Angelina Jolie here. She's so sexy, she's seen as almost scary. Society sets it up so we just can't win.

One last soapbox moment and I'll stop (for now): our culture and the media make it seem like only hot, young, thin, able-bodied people should have sex. The truth is, sex is for everyone, and that includes the elderly, differently abled, obese, not conventionally attractive, bi, gay, trans, nonbinary, straight, skinny, people with ostomies, neurodivergent, and everyone else on Earth. All human beings are inherently sexual beings. (Technically, researchers think 1 to 2 percent of people are truly asexual, but I digress.)

Once you start to see the miseducation women receive and how it affects their relationships with themselves and their partners, you can't unsee it. Understanding and acknowledging how our society treats women and their sexuality is the first step to changing the paradigm. We all have to deal with—and reject—the thoughts that have been instilled in us by society, religion, our families, and people who don't have our best interests at heart. Are you actually fine not touching your clitoris just because somebody told you not to do it in seventh grade?

Break free of wherever that voice came from and make up your own mind what to believe. Be curious. What if there isn't one "right way" to be sexual? What if there's a different way that makes you feel whole, seen, supported, confident, and sexy while receiving or giving pleasure? The answer to all that is inside of you. Let's go there.

The brain is our biggest sex organ, so it has to be included in this equation or everything else is going to fail. Hormones are quite important, but they aren't the holy grail in absentia of everything else. Supplements, self-cultivation, and fancy biodegradable, earth-friendly vibrators (yes, they exist) won't make a difference if we're still thinking the same way about sex. Success will only come when we change our views, what we're worthy of, and what we deserve. We can't enjoy wonderful sex until we take back the power and own our sexuality, ask for what we need, and accept and love ourselves for the miracles we are.

I want you to know it's perfectly okay to feel broken—we come by that easily because of what society tells us—but you didn't get here because you're broken. You got here because of people's unwillingness to tell the truth. I want to help you challenge and throw all those worthless thoughts away and learn new ways of thinking and being. Let's work together to establish a newer, healthier view of sex than the one we received the first time around.

SOCIETAL LIES

We all grew up with "collective belief systems," where a collective belief is adopted by a group as a means to realizing the group's goals. Certainly, our society has goals to control a person's sexuality—especially women. How many of these lies did you learn about sex? How many do you still believe? Hint: none are real, true, or right.

It's time to be more open to what sexuality is. Some of these may still feel very "truthy" to you, but our power is unleashed when we realize these beliefs aren't facts. We are able to become more open, flexible, and let the "fact-y beliefs" go.

1. Heterosexual sex is the "correct way" to have sex.
    a. There is even a "correct way" to have sex.
2. Monogamy is the only way to be in a sexual relationship.
3. "Sex" means penetrative vaginal sex exclusively.
4. Men should be sexual all the time and women are not allowed to be (but then when they aren't, they have low desire and that's a problem, too).
5. Women should save their sexuality for a committed relationship.
6. There are two genders and no spectrum. Each gender needs to conform fully to the way society says they should act (passive sexually, or pursuant sexually).
7. People over fifty don't engage in sex.
8. People with disabilities don't have sex.
9. Women can't—and shouldn't—be too sexual.
10. If women don't want sex, they are frigid.
11. Women should always be available for sex, even if they don't want sex right now.
12. Women don't have their own sexual preferences (they should simply like PIV sex).
13. Women need to "just" sleep with their husbands because they are married (like it is in a job description), even if they don't want to. Saying no results in negative consequences.
14. Teens shouldn't have sex or self-cultivate.

15. Masturbation is bad. Well, but not for men.
16. Two people in a sexual relationship should have the same level of desire.
    a. And the low desire person is the problem.
17. Sexual needs, desires, and fantasies should be stable throughout your life—in other words, what got you off then should get you off now. (Side note: boy, did Ethan Hawke get me desirous in *Reality Bites*, but now that I am a grown-ass woman, I look back at his character and he smoked, was unemployed, and had a completely crappy outlook on life, which is a total current turnoff. But to redeem the actor, Hawke identifies as a feminist and has criticized "the movie business [being] such a boys' club." So circle back to how Hollywood hurts women by depicting sex so poorly and it looks like Mr. Hawke is on our side. Okay, hot again.)
18. Fantasies are bad, abnormal, and dirty.
19. Women should spontaneously desire sex after a long day when they are physically and emotionally drained.
20. You should always want sex more than wanting sleep.
21. You should desire sex in the months to years after having a baby.
22. Having a good sex life is hard.

CHAPTER TWO

"The Rules" Are Ridiculous

I N MEDICAL SCHOOL, one of my professors said to our class, "Fifty percent of what I tell you is going to be wrong—and we don't know what fifty percent that is." He realized he'd been taught things that aren't considered true anymore, and was letting us know the same would undoubtedly happen to us. Science keeps moving forward and making new discoveries, and we were going to have to keep up if we wanted to be the best doctors possible.

So what the heck does that have to do with sex? you might be asking yourself right now. Well, if what you learned about it—from your equally clueless childhood friends, uninformative high school sex ed class, and Hollywood movies—amounts to "the penis goes in the vagina and then the woman orgasms loudly and quickly," it's time to update your knowledge and start operating on some new information.

For instance, I'm going to assume you'll never want to go back to unsatisfying PIV sex now that you know the vast majority of women don't orgasm with PIV sex alone, right? Caveat: if you love the PIV sex you are having, God bless and don't go changing! No-judgment zone. My discussions certainly don't apply to everyone equally.

Let's start by looking at some common "rules" people learn about sex. Check out the reality truth bombs that follow each one—those are the new facts you can use to replace the outdated ideas.

Rule #1: Men know more about sex than women do.

Reality: I hate to be the one to break it to you, but they know just as little as women do and they have the added disadvantage of not owning our parts to practice on. Men weren't offered *How to Please a Woman 101* freshman year of college, just like you didn't take a class on *How to Give a Mind-Blowing Blow Job*. That's why it's important to keep learning together. (Hint: give your partner this book when you're done reading it. Talk about what it taught you. Try new things—repetition is the key to adult learning—and see what new pathways to pleasure open up as a result.)

Rule #2: Sex has to be spontaneous to be enjoyable—we shouldn't schedule it.

Reality: How's that working out for you? I'm sorry, but when you have two busy people, you HAVE to schedule the opportunity for sex. People think that sex was spontaneous when they were dating, but guess what? It was actually scheduled then, too. You had a date on Friday, and that date was going to possibly lead to sex. Sure, you might not have said it out loud, but you both knew, right? Honeymoons are basically scheduled sex. When something matters to us, we prioritize it. Preparing healthy food, scheduling workouts—if we don't make time, these things won't happen. We have to do the same with sex. Without purposefully planning to turn our to-do list off and drop back into our body, it just doesn't automatically happen for a lot of women. To clarify, I am not talking about scheduling sex like a to-do list task. Instead, dedicate time to be close, date, get naked, shower, hold hands, listen. It is about cultivating a sexual/erotic relationship and opportunities to be close, intimate, and erotic, not just "doing PIV" on a timeline.

Rule #3: We shouldn't talk about sex.

Reality: You should talk about sex your entire relationship—it's not a one-and-done kind of conversation. Bodies change, stress changes, appetites change, physical limitations happen. You need to talk about what's going on if you want to keep growing—and sleeping!—together. Sure, it might be awkward in the beginning. Do it anyway. None of us are mind readers. You can't get better at the things you don't work on. And bonus secret: intimacy is created by talking about sex, not just having sex. Vulnerability when shared and received well is sexy as hell. (More on this in Chapter Nine: Communication Is Lubrication.)

Rule #4: Sex starts when the penis goes in the vagina and ends when a man has an orgasm.

Reality: There's a lot more to sex than just putting a penis in a vagina. Things that happen BEFORE the PIV should be called sex (and is by people in the know). PIV sex alone is generally not going to end in you having an orgasm (which is a bummer if it's the only drink on the menu), may even hurt (even worse), and usually starts before the female is adequately aroused. Everything that happens before penetration is just as, if not more, important, ESPECIALLY for women. It gets your pelvis ready to accept a penis. Pelvic arousal (which is blood flow, like an erection) results in more room in the vagina, more cushioning for the tissues, and more lubrication, which is very helpful for the PIV segment of the night, even if you aren't having pain with penetration in the first place. Pro tip: get your pleasure before the P goes in the V. So many people rush to penetrating the vagina and touching sensitive parts before she is ready, which is a turnoff for many women. The mind and body need to be aroused first. Think of arousal on a one to ten scale. If you aren't an eight, don't penetrate.

Rule #5: Pain during sex just comes with the territory.

Reality: Another societal myth tells women the first time is supposed to be painful, which sets us up to think we should just deal with sexual discomfort—even if that extends well beyond losing our virginity (see sidebar for more on this particular word). But here's the thing: sex should not hurt. When it does, premature penetration—putting something inside your body before you're ready for it—and lack of lubrication are commonly to blame. Many of us think, *Oh, the guy is ready, so I should be ready.* Not so! Even though society wants you to think PIV sex is the only kind of sex there is, it's everything that comes BEFORE that makes the vagina ready and willing to accept the penis. An analogy: people just don't go out and sprint. They stretch, do warm-ups, and take a couple of laps around the track before they go all out. Get the body warmed up and ready. The same holds true for the pelvis. If women were just taught not to allow anything in their vagina until they're ready to have something in there, it would revolutionize a lot of people's sex lives. (That being said, see a doctor if you suspect there's some other cause for your pain with sex—it might be due to low estrogen in the vulva, pelvic floor muscle tightness or spasms, vulvodynia, scar or adhesions from surgery or endometriosis, or an infection.) If you have pain with intercourse, don't wonder where your desire for sex went. We don't desire painful stimuli. We avoid it.

Side note: you don't "lose" anything by putting something inside your vagina. Virginity is a social construct, meaning it's a made-up thing. It was created to control women's behavior. According to Radhika Radhakrishnan in her excellent "What Being a Sex-Positive Feminist Means to

Me" essay in *Medium*, "If you've not had specifically penis-in-vagina sex, you're called a 'virgin' which is a patriarchal and heterosexual way of thinking about sex...Virginity is a social construct that commodifies women's bodies...A woman's sexual 'purity' is believed to be attached to her virginity, reducing a woman to her body, her vagina, and giving men immense power over being able to 'transform' women into non-virgins. Such an understanding of sex also erases experiences of lesbian, bisexual, trans women, who are not considered to have 'lost their virginity' unless they've had heterosexual sex with men."[8] Say it louder for the people in the back!

Rule #6: I shouldn't need lube.

Reality: The question should be, why *wouldn't* you need lube? The clitoris and penis don't self-lubricate, and even though the vagina and vulva do, sometimes even that's not enough to make things totally comfortable. Lube makes genital touching and sex WAY more pleasurable. It is actually proven to increase the chance of female orgasm. There are also many circumstances (breastfeeding, perimenopause and menopause, breast cancer, and other cancer treatments) where self-lubrication goes way down. This has nothing to do with how "turned on" you are, so don't make it mean that. Just use lube like an ingredient that is part and parcel to a happy, healthy sex life. An essential oil!

Rule #7: I shouldn't bring toys into the bedroom; it'll be a blow to his ego.

Reality: Toys can be a great way to improve your pleasure—together. They're not meant to replace your partner's penis, fingers, or mouth, but can be used as an enhancement to everything else you're already doing. Using toys isn't a negative judgment of anyone's skills, they're just another tool to ensure a pleasurable time and help level the orgasmic and pleasure playing field. Studies show women who use vibrators in their partnered sex have more satisfied sexual lives.[9] Around 50 percent of women use vibrators, so let's normalize it and jump on the bandwagon of "I'll have what she's having." It is wild to think how much technology we utilize to improve our lives, and this tech was made for your pleasure. We own electric toothbrushes (and now that I am a middle-aged adult, a Waterpik, too) but don't want any technology in our sex lives? Your enjoyment of sex is directly related to your willingness to participate. Willing partner = good times. Enjoy whatever makes you want to show up to the party.

Rule #8: It's not okay if he doesn't orgasm.

Reality: Even the most sexually satisfied couples sometimes have sex that doesn't end in orgasm for one or both partners. Barry McCarthy, in *Rekindling Desire*, says, "even among happily married couples with no history of sexual dysfunction, 5 to 15 percent of sexual encounters are dissatisfying or dysfunctional." That's totally fine. The end goal doesn't always have to be an orgasm. The problem only comes when women think his lack of orgasm means they aren't desirable or sexually skilled enough. Society defines a man's masculinity by his erection and orgasms too, which adds another layer of stress. Sometimes our bodies don't function how we want them to, especially as we age. Erections go away sometimes. Don't add to the stress by making it about you. (PS: if a male orgasm is the very definition of masculinity, then why aren't female orgasm and pleasure the definition of femininity? Double standards abound in the sex world.)

Rule #9: But it IS okay if I don't orgasm (a.k.a. my orgasm isn't as important as his).

Reality: Orgasmic equality matters! Diminishing the importance of the female orgasm diminishes your importance in the sexual relationship. Orgasms are equally available, so of course yours is just as important as your partner's. If half the partnership isn't having as much pleasure and satisfaction, no one should be surprised when that person doesn't want to go to the party as much. Make the party inviting for all people and the party will improve for all.

Rule #10: A woman should only have an orgasm one way—through PIV sex.

Reality: Important things are worth repeating, and after a life of not hearing it this may take a couple of times to sink in: only 20 to 30 percent of women EVER orgasm through PIV sex. Women orgasm much more easily using toys, hands, and mouths, and by focusing on the clitoris. The penis was designed to put sperm in a female close to the uterus—it wasn't designed to be a clitoris expert. But the other body parts that a penis owner owns, oh yeah! So have your orgasm whichever way works for you. Pleasure is the goal. (I will break you from "sex is just PIV" by the end of this book or I have not done my job.)

Rule #11: My partners "give" me orgasms—and if they can't give me one, I'm the problem.

Reality: What feels good to you is your responsibility to find out, and if more people knew what that was, they wouldn't be having rare orgasms and only PIV sex all the time. No one has your exact body or brain and you own the hardware, so start experimenting. Play. Have a blast discovering what gets you going. Then, take responsibility for your own orgasm by communicating your needs to your part-ner. Let's have some compassion here: men also got no training! In general, if you're not having orgasms with him, it's not from a lack of trying—it's from a lack of knowing and communicating what you need. Stop waiting for a man to "give" you an orgasm. Tell or show him what works instead (and that knowledge comes from practice, trial and error, curiosity, and more than one conversation).

Rule #12: All of my orgasms have to be with my partner.

Reality: Um, why? There is no scarcity of orgasms. It's not like, *Oh no, I just used up one of my three orgasms this month by myself! I'm so* *selfish!* You can have as many orgasms as you want with your partner (if they are cool with that). You can also have as many as you want by yourself. You get to decide where, when, and if anyone else is in the room with you. In fact you may even be priming yourself to enjoy sex more, because the data says the more enjoyable sex you have, the more enjoyable sex will be. The more you practice, the faster and more efficient you can be (not that it is about speed). Just saying.

Rule #13: I can't ask for what I want or need because my partner might judge me.

Reality: Communication is essential to a healthy sex life. That's where intimacy is built. The only way ANYONE will ever get what they want and need is by expressing what that is. If you don't know yet, that's okay. Trial and error, listening to feedback, holding space and being vulnerable—all of that is so sexy and totally builds intimacy. Working on your sex life together? Hotness.

Rule #14: My body has to be perfect for me to be a sexual being.

Reality: If you truly believe that sentence, you're taking away the right to be sexual from most of the population. Our habit of self-loathing is often so engrained that we don't even think about it or know it can be changed. EVERY body is worthy of great sex! Stop listening to Hollywood and the media machine. Have at it. You're fine. It may take some work for you, or you can just choose now, SNAP, like that, "I am worthy of having sexuality in my life." The only permission you need is yours (but you have mine too). Your sexual agency does not depend on having a perfect anything. Self-love and nonjudgment will take deliberate practice and attention, but it is work worth doing and there is literally no downside. Cultivating self-love and compassion is very important in this new journey of sexual awareness and awakening into your sexual self, and will spill over in all sorts of beneficial ways outside of the bedroom too. #sexualsideeffects

Rule #15: Men have the right to complain, mope, and be moody until their female partner sleeps with them.

Reality: This may be number one on the list of things that decrease a woman's desire. It is not your job to make him sexually fulfilled all the time, and he is not being an emotional adult—defined as a person who doesn't blame others for the way they feel and act—if he is behaving this way. He is responsible for his behavior, not you. Blaming you isn't cool or sexy, and making it your "job" to have sex with him whenever he wants takes 100 percent of the desire out it. Sex shouldn't be a chore or a job, and when it is, bye-bye desire and enjoyment.

Now what? Write your own rules instead, and when you do, don't let anyone else in your head. Not your ex or your sister or your parents. Not the church. Not society. No one else is going to come to your house and give you self-love and compassion for your body, permission to use toys, block aside time for you to prioritize your pleasure, or communicate with your partner for you. Decide what works for you as a couple and don't pay any mind to what someone might have told you in the past was "right" and "wrong." Right and wrong don't even exist when it comes to sex. Consensual sex is one rule that should always be followed, as well as a pleasurable experience for all involved. The "right" and "wrong" after that is up to you—not the fake rules we just reviewed.

Remember when you were a little kid and you didn't care what anybody thought about you? Cultivate that state of mind when it comes to sex. My goal is for all women to stop giving their sexual power to someone else. It is inherently yours. You have everything you need.

Even if you haven't expressed your sexuality in years, it's still there. You can come back to it at any time. All that takes is getting a little more curious and playful. Have fun with it! It is a journey—there is no "there" to get to. The journey and exploration are the whole point. I coached a woman in her seventies to reexplore her sexuality with her long-term partner. She cried after the work she was able to do after decades of not being intimate. You are never too old or too anything! If you don't give yourself permission, no therapist, lube, toy, hormone supplement, loving partner, or tantric breathing is going to do it for you. Your own permission is THAT essential.

All thoughts can be questioned, and if you think yours can't because somehow your thought is a "belief," know that beliefs are just thoughts you've thought so many times before that they feel real. I call these thoughts "fact-y thoughts," which is cute and, for me at least, takes away their power of "fact."

Finding yours helps pinpoint what may be holding you back in your sexual journey, and writing them down is better than trying to think this out because #neuroscience. It's how the brain works. Trust me, this is important work worth doing.

What are your rules and beliefs about sex?

Who or what taught them to you (implicitly or explicitly)?

Are these rules serving you well or holding you back?

Finally, fill in the blanks.

People who have enjoyable sex:

Thoughts that are preventing me from enjoying sex are:

The ancient Stoic philosophers offer that the obstacle is the way. So the things that are preventing you from enjoying your true sexual self are showing you exactly the work that needs to be done.

CHAPTER THREE

Bad Sex Sucks

A PATIENT RECENTLY CONFIDED in me that her sex life with her ex-husband consisted of him "pounding" her their entire twenty-plus-year marriage. What a nightmare! I imagined her lying there completely disassociated from her body while he had PIV sex with her, not caring (and never asking) whether she was getting any pleasure out of the experience. No wonder she still had pain and fear—and no pleasure—during sex.

Now divorced, in her fifties, and entering a new relationship, she wanted to make her own pleasure a priority. I sent her to a skilled pelvic floor therapist to help her understand her anatomy and conditioned responses. She worked hard to shed her negative associations to sex and is now—for the very first time in her life—enjoying being intimate with her new partner.

That's an extreme example for sure, but I hear these stories all the time and the point is: maybe it's not that you don't enjoy sex. Maybe it's simply that you're having BAD sex. Sex that isn't serving you. It is something done TO you instead of something that is FOR you.

Think of it this way. I love chocolate chip mint ice cream, Häagen-Dazs specifically. I absolutely cannot get enough of it...UNLESS it's melted. Then there's not a chance I want to eat it. I do not desire warm, melted ice cream in the least bit. You can't give me a pill or serve it up in a fancy bowl with a vibrating spoon to make me like it. Nothing will work. Sex, like ice cream, has to be good enough to be WORTH desiring. Sex researcher Peggy Kleinplatz, PhD, wonders why "so many people think they ought to feel 'sexual' desire in the absence of sex worth wanting."

So What Is Bad Sex?

No one wants or desires bad sex, which I define as:

- **Having sex to match your partner's libido when you don't want to.** Research shows it's extremely rare for couples to have the exact same sex drive. So if you're having more sex than you'd like because you think having a different libido than your partner is a problem, know there is no standard anyone has to meet. Negotiate a plan with your partner that will make everyone happy enough instead. The point here is if you are eating more ice cream because your partner wants ice cream, it may explain your growing distaste for ice cream—which you used to love, when you had control over the portion size. More of a good thing isn't always a good thing—for sex and food and pleasurable stuff in general. (More on how to deal with desire mismatch later.)
- **Mercy sex.** Do you find yourself having sex because your partner "needs" it and you figure, *That's what a wife supposed to do?* Women are socialized to think our worth is based on what we do for others, which often leads to having sex when we really aren't into it. It is easy to think we are doing a good

thing, but mercy sex retrains you to resent your partner and sex and numb out until it's over. If any of this sounds like you, please stop saying yes when you mean no. This is how sex becomes an obligation, and one way that genital touch becomes disassociated with pleasure. Sadly, I see this scenario all the time and often it isn't addressed.

- **Checklist sex.** This is when you add sex to the overwhelming list of things to do in your head and it becomes a chore. Dishes, check. Kids all tucked in, check. It's been a week since we had sex so we better do it today, check. Checklist sex turns intimacy into a "should" instead of a pleasure, and that is definitely NOT sexy.

Consent means agreeing to have sex. Most women having mercy or checklist sex are perhaps TECHNICALLY agreeing—they aren't saying no. But they also really aren't saying yes. Or maybe they feel like they CAN'T say no, which is the same as not having agency. An important part of consent is the ability to say no without any negative consequences. Conversations about consent need to become part of sex education and reinforced to all genders often so fewer people end up in this situation.

- **Coercive sex or using sex as a bartering chip in a relationship.** If your partner always gets to decide when it's going to happen and you have no say in it, that's a hard no. Forced sexual intercourse is NEVER okay—this is called intimate partner violence. On the flip side, withholding sex because you're angry and want to punish your partner isn't healthy, either. Good sex isn't one-sided and doesn't have those kinds of strings attached. True story: one woman would collect a "point" from her husband each time she had sex with him, which she could then redeem for things. Guess what, she had little interest in sleeping with him. Who would?

- **Accepting that pain is involved.** Be sure to spend enough time on your arousal (a.k.a. foreplay) or activities that focus on getting blood flow and good feelings into the female pelvis before you jump into the PIV part. Like I said in the last chapter, a very common nonmedical cause of pain during sex is premature penetration and lack of adequate lubrication. Don't put anything in your vagina until you're ready. That can go a long way in making it pleasurable instead of painful. (If that doesn't do it, see your doctor to find out if something else is causing the issue.) I once saw a woman who occasionally had pain and bleeding after sex. When I asked her when it happened, she said during rougher sex without enough foreplay and lube. Yup, nailed it. Your body needs to get ready.

- **Faking orgasms.** Have you ever faked it because you just wanted the sex to end? I hate to be the bearer of bad news, but all that does is set up a positive feedback loop for bad sex. Your partner thinks, *I'm going to repeat what I did last time because it worked so well!* while you're stuck thinking, *But I did that because it WASN'T working well!* Some women believe men are to blame here; if the guy had just "given" them an orgasm, they wouldn't have to fake it. That would be nice to hear—it's all the man's fault!—but you're an active player in this charade and you're going to have to take responsibility for that. Ask for what you want and you'll get what you need more regularly. (Also a quick aside here: intimacy without orgasm is fine—that's not bad sex. There are plenty of sexually satisfied couples where sometimes it just doesn't work for one or the other party. You can still enjoy being with each other and have some fun.)

- **Wanting—but not having—orgasms.** A lot of women tell me, "Sure, it would be nice to have an orgasm, but it usually doesn't happen." Do you think a guy would go into a sexual experience with a meh, *whatever happens, happens* attitude like that? Not typically! Stop selling that part of the experience short. Talk to your partner about what's going to get you there. Better yet, show them. This is the part where you need the self-cultivation skills to gain this useful knowledge and the communication skills to discuss what your body needs.

- **When the woman's orgasm isn't valued as much as the man's.** This all goes back to the patriarchal view of sex, how PIV is society's entire definition of sex, and how that ends in male orgasm with no regard for a woman's fulfillment. We've been sold a bill of goods that we're "complicated" and "difficult" in terms of our orgasms, but honestly, is spending time focusing on the clitoris and paying equal attention to both people's pleasure so radical? It may be a culture change for you and your partner, but it is one that is good for everyone.

- **PIV sex only.** Let's face it: if that's all you're doing, your partner is probably not going to last long enough to make you orgasm and you'll just "numb out" because you're not adequately aroused. Not to mention, often you are not receiving enough clitoral stimulation during the act to get you there no matter how Herculean the effort is. The movies and sex ed told us this is what sex is, but studies show up to 70 percent of women don't orgasm this way so it's time to put it on the "bad sex" list. I recently mentioned my theory of "maybe it's just bad sex" to a male colleague who researches low desire. He replied, "Of course women should be having good sex!" It led me to believe that he thinks all women with low desire are having fantastic sex when they have it—like that's the assumed default. This is a very male-centric viewpoint to assume women have the same kind of great sex men usually experience—and so many women have shared with me that they are not.

BTW, I'm not trying to throw shade at men here. I love men! Sex is the only thing we're all supposed to be experts in, but none of us ever got any training. We have to work together to make things better! He doesn't have our parts and didn't get any better education than we did. You have to help him along here. Just as it is not your fault, it is not his fault either.

According to psychologist and sex educator Barry McCarthy, good sex adds 15 to 20 percent additional value to a relationship. Bad or nonexistent sex drains it by an estimated 50 to 70 percent, and when sex "provokes conflict, it takes on an inordinately powerful role, destabilizing the relationship."[10] That means bad sex is far worse for a relationship than good sex is good for one. As an active player in your sex life, you need to own where you are in all this and make an effort to correct it. Hope is not a strategy.

Bad sex really just comes down to a giant miscommunication between partners, our bodies, and society's miseducation of what heterosexual sex should be. Reeducating both people in a relationship and expanding the view of what sex is to accommodate women's needs and pleasure is the solution.

What about Good Sex?

Good sex is when your pleasure is as important as your partner's. When foreplay—everything leading up to penetration—is at least as much of the show, if not far more, than the PIV itself. When your pleasure is achieved the way that works best for you. It's intimacy and enjoying your partner, your time together, mutual pleasure, and genital touch.

It's also about enjoying your body, which, may I remind you once again, has a clitoris you carry around with you twenty-four seven. So many women have body image issues that stop them from having fun in bed. They think they're too jiggly or soft, or that their breasts are too small or too big or droopy or veiny. It is time to start working on this, because it truly doesn't matter what your body looks like. It's a body. It is yours. Sonya Renee Taylor, in her amazing book *The Body Is Not an Apology*, talks about building a radical self-love practice in an age of loathing.

If you want to be a porn star, you might have to look a certain way, but if you just want to have an orgasm in your bedroom, nobody cares. (And if your partner cares, maybe you need to reevaluate the partner—because it turns out, most men see beauty where we see flaws. They are simply happy we are naked and playing with them.)

Research shows that women who have more body confidence— which is far more about your THOUGHTS than your LOOKS— enjoy their sex lives more and are more sexually active. *So how do I get body confidence?* you might ask. *Buy something?* No. The only thing you have to do is decide that you have it. No one and nothing else can give it to you. The power is truly inside you. Start seeing the thoughts (reminder that thoughts aren't facts) that are negative as just ANTs (automatic negative thoughts), which are a normal function of all brains. See them, say hi, then work to let them go and release their power by not "grasping" on to them.

Judging yourself is a waste of energy that would be better spent on other things. Check in with your values. How does self-loathing and body shaming align with them? Perfection wreaks havoc on our body image and sex life.

This is the body you have right now. It is present, in front of you. Ready for your love. Stop waiting for someone else to give you permission to feel good about yourself. This may take some work after years of talking negatively to yourself, but it is some of the best work you can do for yourself, your children, and your relationship. You truly have more love to give when you love yourself. Enlist a coach or a therapist if you need to.

Would you ever body-shame someone else? No! Shame is always based on a lie. Shame is the belief that something is wrong with you. Shame researcher Brené Brown says, "Where perfectionism exists, shame is always lurking."

Body confidence comes from your mind, not the size of your body. You think you need to be more disciplined in eating and exercising, but you actually just need to be more disciplined in the way you are thinking.

Our brains are designed with a negativity bias. It helped keep us alive in the caves of yesteryear. But now negative thoughts don't keep us safe as much as they hold us back. There is zero benefit in beating yourself up. If beating yourself up worked, all women would be thin and tall, with perfect hair and skin and and and...stop it!

Here's another secret: if you don't love yourself as you are now, it is unlikely you will love yourself when you are thinner, fitter, older, or whatever else you think the goal may be. Say "no thank you" to thinking about yourself negatively.

This is my body. Be in that space. Acceptance. Then radical self-love.

Coming full circle here: maybe you don't actually have the problem you thought you had. Maybe this has nothing to do with you not liking sex very much. Maybe it's just bad sex you don't like and therefore don't desire.

No one wants melted ice cream—so let's learn how to have the frozen, decadent, delicious kind instead, as an active participant, when you are ready and interested in it. Onward!

Dr. Barry McCarthy has also developed the idea of Good-Enough Sex, which is pretty awesome. It offers a commonsense yet comprehensive perspective that challenges our notions of sex and encourages couples to pursue positive, realistic meaning in their intimate lives. "With the Good-Enough Sex model, intimacy is the ultimate focus, with pleasure as important as function, and mutual emotional acceptance as the environment. Sex is integrated into the couple's daily life and daily life is integrated into their sex life to create the couple's unique sexual style. Living daily life well—with its responsibilities, stresses, and conflicts—provides the opportunity to experience sexual interactions in a subtly yet distinctively personalized and enriched way. Sex at times is experienced as pleasure, stress relief, mature playfulness, and on another occasion as a spiritual union. Intimate couples can value multiple purposes for sex and use several styles of arousal. Good-Enough Sex recognizes that among satisfied couples the quality of sex varies from day to day and from very good to mediocre or even dysfunctional. Such reasonable expectations are an important feature of sexual satisfaction as well as inoculating the couple from disappointment and sexual problems in the future."[11] Preach!

PART TWO:

Sex-Positive Sex Ed for Adults

CHAPTER FOUR

The Female Edition

REMEMBER THAT SCENE in the 2004 movie *Mean Girls* where the full extent of Coach Carr's sex ed class was *Don't have sex, because you will get pregnant and die! Don't have sex in the missionary position, don't have sex standing up, just don't do it, okay, promise? Okay, now everybody take some rubbers.* If your formal education came from a high school teacher who sounded a lot like Coach Carr, it's time for some better information.

Sex ed in this country is woefully lacking and fear-based. "Highlights" include:

1. Just don't do it.
2. How NOT to get pregnant or a sexually transmitted infection (STI).
3. That guys have a penis, and women only have internal organs like the ovaries, uterus, and vagina.

4. Sex is when the penis goes in the vagina and nothing else (which is so heteronormative, not to mention incredibly limiting even for those of us who are heterosexual. It is very rare that same-sex, bisexual, or nongender-conforming sex gets talked about at all.)

5. How to put a condom on a banana. Maybe. If you're lucky.

Preventing pregnancy and infection are important—but that's just one small facet of a much larger and far more complex subject. Teaching sex ed by saying, "Don't get pregnant or diseases" is like telling a chef, "Don't use moldy lettuce." That's not how you learn to cook well.

Tell me...did you hear anything about the clitoris and vulva during sex ed? And if by some miracle it got mentioned, did you learn that it's the female equivalent of a penis in terms of pleasure? My guess is NO. And it's almost certain you didn't hear sex explained from the female-dominant perspective—that the penis is the male clitoris.

So why is it okay to teach people how to put on condoms, but not teach where the clitoris is or that it's the female organ of pleasure? Or that people have sex because it is pleasurable? *Why are you teenagers having sex? Oh, we're just practicing not getting pregnant!*

Or maybe, like me, you went to a school where sex ed didn't even exist (Catholic school through sixth grade for this woman right here). The scant information I got wasn't going to be much help unless I wanted to stay celibate for life. The most important female was a virgin and had a kid without even putting a P in the V. And if I, unlike her, was actually going to have sex, it had to happen after marriage and be for procreation, not pleasure.

In 2018, a record 35 percent of Americans between twenty-five and fifty had never been married, so "saving it for marriage" excludes many adults as well. What's more, according to The Knot, the average age of marriage in the United States is currently thirty-one for a female and thirty-three for men. Is an entire generation of humans supposed to wait thirteen years after becoming a legal adult to have sex? That's completely unrealistic.

We need more sex education, not less. The fact that we are so completely incapable of even talking about the topic (doctors included) tells me this is exactly what we need to be talking about. Given the current lack of education, though, it's not surprising that most people don't know what the term sex-positive means. The Oxford English Dictionary defines it as *having or promoting an open, tolerant, or progressive attitude towards sex and sexuality*. Basically, it means telling the good side of the story, and it's actually a very cool way to talk about sex. I didn't even hear the term "sex-positive" until a few years ago, and I fell in love with it.

You probably didn't get a sex-positive education if you learned about sex from porn, your friend's dad's *Playboy* magazine (or gay porn in my case), or Hollywood movies. Those are not often accurate portrayals. You are watching fiction—and commonly fiction made for what works for the male mind and body. It's like learning how to drive from the *Fast & Furious* movie franchise. Technically driving, but not applicable to many people with cars.

My mother was very modern in many ways, and taught me feminism, told me I could do and be anything I wanted in my life, and pushed me to go to medical school when my own self-doubt clouded my thinking. She made us use the correct words for body parts and their functions. Not until much later did I realize how unique and helpful this was—like when a father called his four-year-old's vulva her "taco" when I was doing pediatric urology, or when my recent sixty-five-year-old female in clinic said she had a problem with her "hoo-ha." Social media continues to play a part in this by banning anatomically correct words for female body parts. They are effectively erased. Nonexistent. Dirty and bad and forbidden. When we take away the words for our pelvic structures, we eliminate a common vocabulary needed to communicate with our sexual partner and doctors in times of illness or pain.

Unfortunately, my parents weren't much more illuminating than the church with regard to sex. I guess that's why I was so curious about it when I was growing up. Like many of us, I heard it was going to hurt, but there were certainly never any conversations like, "Let's talk about how to make your first time comfortable and on your own terms."

Once, when I was home from college on a break and my family went out for pizza, I remember my parents asking me when I thought they should talk to my high-school-aged brothers about sex. (Oh, so NOW they wanted to talk about it?) All I could say was, "Yeah, it's too late. They're already having sex—or at least they're trying to." (I didn't actually know what they were up to, but I still knew it was too late.)

A patient in her eighties recently told me that when she first got her period at twelve, on Christmas Day, she had no clue what was going on so she asked her mother. Her mom told her, "You have the curse. If you get pregnant, we'll disown you." This poor little child had no idea what menstruation was, let alone how to get pregnant or avoid pregnancy—yet all she heard was that she was cursed and could be expelled from her own family!

When basic body functions are considered shameful and humiliating, it only follows that sex becomes a problem. On a side note, I am frequently reminded by my patients' stories that we all walk around as adults but are really just "grown-up children" living in a world that we learned to interpret via our family from a very young age. The culture we come from is the culture we live, repeat, and pass on unless we take the time to see it for what it is, challenge it, and change the narrative.

It's no wonder so many women suffer such shame and guilt about sex. No wonder we flounder around, using whatever information we've picked up from less-than-helpful sources, hoping to get it right. I don't think that's going well for most people, so let's take a look at what's REALLY happening with our bodies.

How Female Bodies Work

For starters: not everything "down there" is your vagina. Vulva is actually the correct term for the female genitalia you can see. This includes the labia majora and minora—a.k.a. the outer and inner lips—plus the clitoris and the urethral and vaginal opening to the hymen. This non-hair-bearing skin area of the vulva at the entrance of the vagina is called the vestibule.

> The hymen shares a name origin with the Greek god Hymen, son of Apollo, who was the wedding god. Hymen means to join, referring to how the vagina forms embryo-logically. One theory why the hymen exists (because Mother Nature isn't talking) is that it decreases infection. (Ever change a baby girl's poopy diaper and wonder why she doesn't get an infection? Could be the hymen protection.)
>
> Many vagina-owning mammals have a hymen and the idea that it evolved because males prefer virgins is down-right harmful. Ob-gyn Jonathan Schaffir says, "The idea that virginity can be measured or verified (from a hymen exam) is perhaps the most harmful and damaging myth. Assuming that a woman's sexual behavior can be inferred from her appearance is demeaning..."[12] Agree.

The name vagina stems from a Latin word for sheath, as in to sheath a sword. This is just another example of the male default, naming women's body parts for the service it provides men. Depending on what research you're looking at, the average adult vagina measures between 3.7 to 4.5 inches and lengthens with arousal.[13] The average erect penis is about 5.25 inches long according to a 2015 study (you needed this info, I know).[14] That means, on average—again, this is all averages—the unaroused vagina is 33 percent shorter than the average erect penis size. Arousal—blood flow and muscle relaxation—can expand the vagina by double or triple the unaroused capacity. An aroused vagina tips back, getting the cervix and uterus out of the way. Arousal is key to pain prevention with penetration. If it isn't an eight, don't penetrate! Have I mentioned lately repetition is the key to adult learning?

Even with giving full consent, truly wanting to have sex, and having adequate clitoral stimulation to lengthen the average vagina to accommodate the average penis, a penis (or a toy) may still be too big and hurt. A cool tool for length discrepancy mismatch is the "oh nut," which is a bit like a stackable silicone innertube to use as a bumper against too much length (it is also good for vaginas shortened by surgery or radiation).[15]

Moving on: the clitoris is the female version of a penis. The glans, or external part of the clitoris, is less than 20 percent of its actual anatomy. The freely movable skin over the glans, called the clitoral hood, is the equivalent of the foreskin in males. Behind that, there's the shaft, or body, of the clitoris, which is analogous to the shaft of the penis and is still considered an outside structure. If you rub your fingers back and forth between the mons pubis (the fleshy part on your pubic bone) and the clitoral glans, you're feeling your clitoral body! From there, the clitoris basically breaks into two parts like a wishbone, curving underneath the labia and pelvic bone on both sides. This is equivalent to the corpus cavernosum—two channels of tissue that run the length of the penis—in male anatomy. If you tap the lateral walls inside your vagina, you are actually tapping on the clitoral bulbs. These are why vaginal penetration works well for some women—because the stretch, fullness, and friction stimulates the erectile tissue of the clitoral bulbs.

I'm going to be honest here, I didn't learn any of this in surgery training or medical school. I only found out when a sex therapist showed me a 3-D model of the clitoris a few years back. At the time, I remember thinking, *That can't be right. I would've learned that if it was right!* Take that one in: I made it through medical school. I operate in the pelvis. Yet it's like our entire organ of pleasure doesn't really exist! So if you have no idea what the structure actually looks like or how it works, you are most definitely not alone, even if you are a medical doctor.

I guess it doesn't matter that none of this made it into the med school curriculum anyhow, because nearly all the available information about clitoral anatomy is incorrect. For instance, the clitoral body (shaft) and the clitoral nerves—which are each two to three millimeters in diameter and travel the entire length of the clitoral body before reaching the glans—are way longer than most textbooks imply. Just to get super science geeky on you here: "The clitoral body is substantial in length, mostly lying superficially under the clitoral hood and mons pubis. The dorsal nerves of the clitoris are large and superficial, terminating at or near the base of the clitoral glans...The mean length of the descending clitoral body, from the angle to the base of the glans, was 37.0 mm."[16] The clitoris is nearly the size of a penis, but no one is told this so our organ of pleasure gets diminished in anatomy texts, sex ed, and in real life.

Are you imagining only the glans at the twelve o'clock position on the vulva as the clitoris? Most people think that, but it's really just the tip of the iceberg. The clitoris also includes the shaft and the bulbs that lie under your labia. The whole area around your entrance to the vagina—called the vestibule—contains erectile tissue, which is why labial massage and vibration can feel so good. Understanding this anatomy and erectile/arousal tissue also helps you understand why the penis isn't the best object to stimulate female orgasms. It isn't great at bringing blood flow to the erectile tissues of the clitoral complex surrounding the vagina. In our practice of expanding the previously narrow PIV definition of sex to include pleasant sexual touch, please consider stimulating ALL of the clitoris and vulva as "sex" going forward. Touching the body in general, moving inward towards the pelvis, can be much more effective at turning on a female body. Going straight to the vagina is jarring and a turn-off for many people.

Have you ever heard or read the fact that the clitoris has eight thousand nerve endings? Sounds super legit until you discover that information comes from a livestock study done on COWS. We don't take any of our other health information from cows, so just saying, it's insulting. If women are going to be taught how many nerve endings our clitoris has, it should at least be from a human study (which hasn't been done yet to my knowledge).

With sexual stimulation, the sympathetic nervous system brings blood flow to the vulva, clitoris, and vagina. The temperature of the genitals increases. Secretions, which make things feel better and protect our tissues from the friction and injury of sexual activity, lubricate the vulva and vagina.

These secretions are a combination of mucin released from androgen-dependent glands of the vulva (Bartholin's, Skene's, and minor vestibular glands) and transudate of blood serum that leaks through aquaporins channels in the vaginal mucosa—sort of like sweating. Yup, it's true. Vaginal moisture is basically sweat.

As the genitals become engorged with blood, the labia gets bigger. The vagina lengthens and tips back, and the pelvic floor muscles relax and become more accommodating so penetration can happen without pain. The nipples may harden and become erect; the skin flushes; and heart rate, blood pressure, and the breath increase.

With enough clitoral stimulation and your mind staying in your body and on sexy thoughts instead of the grocery list, orgasm usually occurs in twenty to thirty minutes with a partner, or just a few if you're self-cultivating. Basically, an orgasm is a release of muscle tension at 0.8 second intervals (yes, people measure this stuff). In 1953, Kinsey defined orgasm as "the expulsive discharge of neuromuscular tension at the peak of sexual response." In 1966, Masters and Johnson said it was "a brief episode of physical release from the vasocongestion and muscle tension developed in response to sexual stimuli." I say those are very unsexy descriptions of something that feels incredibly amazing (more about how to optimize your orgasms later). Summary: orgasm = a buildup and then a release.

When people talk about the G-spot—an area on the anterior vaginal wall that's sensitive and pleasurable to women—what's actually being stimulated is the body/shaft of the clitoris from the inside of the vagina, as well as the corpora spongiosum (erectile tissue surrounding the urethral opening called the clitoral-urethral complex). Yes, women have erectile tissue— same as penis owners—and paying attention to those structures is important for a woman's pleasure, enjoyment, and desire for sex. Some call the area the female prostate. Bottom line: the G-spot is not so much a "spot" as it is a "region of interest."

As Betty Dodson, PhD, sexologist, and proponent of women's sexual pleasure and health for over four decades, explains, "There is no distinction between 'vaginal' or 'clitoral' or 'G-spot' orgasms since all orgasms are centered in the clitoris. A woman's erection takes twenty to thirty minutes of adequate clitoral stimulation for her entire vulva to become engorged." If it takes less, not a problem; if it takes more, not a problem. Why oh why are we in such a hurry?

An Education on Lubrication

The amount of natural lubrication a woman's body produces is often not an indication of how "hot" she is for sex. Women can have desire and not enough moisture, and conversely, have moisture and not want sex. Her level of moisture has nothing to do with how into sex she is. Wetness or lack of it doesn't prove anything. Time and again I see men pressure women to "be more wet" or tell them they are or aren't turned on because of their moisture level. It's not an on-demand faucet, women can't consciously control it, and pressuring women or assuming intent from her moisture isn't sexy at all.

We can want sex and not feel like we have enough lubrication. The experts call this arousal desire mismatch or nonconcordance (disagreement between mind and body), and it is quite common and not even considered a problem or pathologic. Research shows that discordance is more common in heterosexual women, while in men, the erection and brain are more synchronized and erection = I want to have sex. But again, men have nonconcordance too, especially in the early years when the wind blowing can cause an erection (as in, his penis is erect but he doesn't want sex at that time). Data shows mindfulness can help increase concordance. Some of the woo-woo stuff is super helpful for sex.

Medications, chronic health conditions, age, and hormones can all affect the amount of secretions we make. Menopause, breastfeeding, and the time of the month for menstruating women all factor in there as well. Spend your attention on female genital touch, vibration, or whatever gets you most wet, and/or use lube, but don't obsess over your level of vaginal sweat.

Besides, even if you are producing enough moisture, the clitoris does not self-lubricate, which is why lube is one of God's gifts to the modern world. Eighty percent of women say having an orgasm is easier when they use lube. Believe me when I tell you that people having good sex use lube. Some people think if you don't have a towel down during sex, you're doing it wrong!

Yes, even young people need lube. I had a twenty-two-year-old woman consult with me for pain with sex. It turns out, she and her boyfriend were just putting the penis in the vagina. That's it—the extent of what they did together. They weren't using lube because her boyfriend told her she shouldn't need it. That's freaking tragic, but even more tragic is that she made it all the way to a surgeon when the only thing she needed was some education (and maybe some lube, but maybe not—maybe she just needed some clitoral and vulvar stimulation before putting the P in the V, allowing her body to prepare for penetration). Crappy sex ed strikes again.

Make sure your lube is condom-friendly if you use condoms, and sperm-friendly if you are trying to conceive. As a general rule, silicone-based lubes are best in show because they don't get absorbed into our tissues, which makes them last longer, especially with dry skin, menopause, and in trans men (high "male" level testosterone causes dry vaginas). Water-based lube is recommended when using silicone toys. Coconut oil is good in a pinch but not with condoms, and not if you are prone to infections (it is a food).

FYI, experts hate KY Jelly. It has a "tacky" feeling and high osmolality—basically, it draws moisture from your cells into the product, causing skin irritation and dehydration. The World Health Organization actually has a lube guideline of less than 1200mOsm/kg (lower than KY and Astroglide) and a pH of around 4.5 (natural pH of the vagina) so as to not cause infection or irritation. You can find a ton of different options—flavors, scents, and sensations produced (don't use these if sensitive or prone to infection)—online and at sexual health stores, so don't feel like you have to settle for that basic bitch of lubes at your local drugstore. Experiment! Get some good stuff. I like the two silicone brands, Über Lube and Gun Oil.

Get Aroused!

We obviously know how to tell when a guy is aroused. He gets an erection, and then he's ready to penetrate the vagina. Women have very similar amounts of erectile tissue in the clitoris as men do in the penis, and we need to be aroused before having sex or it will not be enjoyable. We usually don't try to stuff a flaccid penis in there, right? Well, it's the same idea with women.

When we're aroused, sex is fun and orgasms can happen. Without arousal, pain, dryness, mental wandering, distraction, and decreased ability to orgasm happen. Lack of arousal is one reason why so many women feel dissociated or "numb" down there. This is why it's so important to avoid premature penetration.

For women, pelvic arousal is brought on by the vascular system and nervous system. Female genital arousal is a physical state arising from processing physical (touch) and nonphysical (thoughts) stimuli, leading to increased activity in the central and peripheral nervous systems.

These two types of arousal are referred to as genital and nongenital or emotional (the latter two referring to originating in the brain). Genital arousal is when the genitals change in response to sexual stimuli. Nongenital arousal happens when there is positive mental engagement and focus in response to a sexual stimulus.

Just to be clear, arousal is different from desire. Desire is a *wanting* for sex, and can come AFTER arousal. In fact, desire doesn't need to happen at all to have wonderful sex (more on that in Chapter Eleven: Desire Is So Two-Faced).

Arousal is higher to novel stimuli—that is, new things—because our brains are PAYING ATTENTION. This is also why the "same old, same old" tends to feel less exciting over time. For instance, the more you watch the same sexually charged movie, the LESS aroused you get. Novelty also increases dopamine, which is where desire comes from. You won't desire activities that don't give you a nice dose of dopamine, so work on great arousal and sex to stoke your desire. It is the anticipatory feedback loop and neuroscience. Switch things up! Keep it fresh! We get in a rut with sex and then want it less as a result of it not being novel to our brain. Stereotypically, women need more novelty and variety with their sexuality. Stereotypically, men can do the same-old-works-for-years style of sex without fail. Some say this is because women have more active brain connections. Whatever the reason, there's nothing wrong with you if you don't desire boring, repetitive sex.

Focus on the now, your body (all of it, moving inward to the genitals, not just wham bam vagina), and its sensations to increase arousal. This is a learned behavior and you will get better at it with practice. Magnificent sex is never a passive accident!

Distracting, nonerotic thoughts during sex, like feeling unattractive and pressure to perform, also decrease arousal. Watching yourself proverbially having sex or "being the watcher" is called "spectatoring" and it is not where pleasure and orgasm live. Chronic and acute stress dampen arousal as well. Take a good look at those kinds of issues before jumping to the conclusion that you have some sort of a physical problem getting aroused.

So that's it: factually correct sex ed about women's bodies. Way better than the job Coach Carr did in *Mean Girls*, right?

It would be easy to believe that sex ed has improved a million percent since we were growing up. That parents teach their kids all the facts we've already talked about here, plus everything that's yet to be learned (I know I am still learning about sex all the time). That young people someday will not make it to my office complaining of pain with sex because they know premature penetration without lube is poor form when you are trying to please a woman as equally as a man.

Sadly, that's not the case. I see my fair share of uninformed millennials and Gen Z-ers who weren't taught anything more than we were—not in school and not by their parents. In fact, they may even be worse off than us, because porn has been their main teacher.

Porn has contributed to an influx of college-aged guys showing up at mental health clinics confused about why sex isn't anything like what they see on their screens. Why doesn't their penis look and work like that? Why is real sex so AWKWARD? What are they supposed to do with their feelings?

Porn is the reason young women wonder why they aren't flailing their legs and screaming in ecstasy the second a penis goes in their vagina. Is their body broken? Are THEY broken? Is everyone just supposed to act and fake it?

It's time to stop this cycle of miseducation before it goes any further. How? We need to start speaking the truth to our kids and anyone else looking to us for advice. Let's get REAL about REAL sex. And bonus if we can start talking about it like the weather—it is common, ever-changing, sometimes pleasant, sometimes not. Porn isn't going away, but using it for sex ed can.

Here are some pointers to get us going:

Use proper words. It's a vulva, clitoris, and vagina. It's a penis and scrotum. You pee (okay you got me, urinate) out of the urethra. There are plenty of studies showing that kids who use proper words are more likely to speak up in cases of sexual misconduct, and people are more likely to believe them because they use the correct terminology. Also, people can communicate with their doctor better when things are amiss. This is empowerment.

Boundaries are important. If you don't want to hug somebody, you don't have to. If you don't want to kiss someone, don't. You don't need to give an explanation. You have power over your body no matter what age you are. Consent must be part of the conversation. It is mandatory. Communication, respect, and honesty are part of a good relationship. When you don't want to have sex, no means no. No doesn't mean, "until he can convince me."

Self-cultivation/masturbation is not dirty. We're all sexual beings, and it's not bad to touch yourself. It feels good for a reason, because we are born that way. Having orgasms can relieve stress, assist in sleep, and decrease pain among other benefits, so have at it in the privacy of your own bedroom. Your body is not "to be saved" for someone else. It is yours.

Respect others. We're all living, breathing human beings—not just bodies. People aren't objects to be obtained or used for sex.

It's not okay unless you say it's okay. Nothing sexual happens unless everyone consents to it. Only participate if you want to, not because you think someone else wants you to. (It's also a good idea to add a side conversation here about why alcohol is so dangerous to boundaries and sexual consent.)

Use proper protection. Getting all the facts about birth control and using it properly leads to better sex knowing pregnancy and STIs have been prevented as best they can up front.

Sex is to be enjoyed. It is one of life's biggest pleasures. It is not dirty or shameful, and should never be painful.

Both partners get equal pleasure. Sex is about figuring out how to make each other feel good together. Find out what your partner wants and what makes them feel good. Orgasmic equality is where it's at.

Don't practice premature penetration. Women's genitals need to be erect and engorged before PIV sex just like men's do. This requires paying attention to the clitoris and vulva as well as mental stimulation before penetration. If women are not physically and mentally aroused, it's not time for PIV sex yet.

Orgasm from PIV sex is rare. The female equivalent to the penis is the clitoris, not the vagina, and it does not typically get enough stimulation from PIV sex alone for orgasm. Pay attention to the clitoris first using hands, mouths, or toys before penetrating. Change the heterosexual narrow paradigm that PIV sex is the only kind of sex!

Communication makes sex better. Other countries are much better at teaching teenagers about communication, navigating conversations about what to do if one person doesn't want to wear a condom, and the ever-necessary topic of consent. We have a long way to go to prepare the future generations for communicating well about sex. Talking about sex in the beginning of a relationship is key—because the longer you wait, the harder it gets. Don't assume someone should know how to turn you on, or that you automatically know how to turn someone on without asking. We don't all like the same things. What worked with your last partner might not with the next one.

You're completely normal. The message here is don't worry. I can't tell you how many older women I've seen in my clinic who say, "I wish someone had told me everything I was experiencing was totally normal. It would have saved me from so much guilt, shame, and doubt." Let's save the next generation from this kind of fear when it comes to sex.

CHAPTER FIVE

The Male Edition

YOU MIGHT BE surprised to learn that it's not only women who get the shaft—pun intended—from society when it comes to sex. Men also have a bunch of harsh expectations put on them. They're told they need to have a high sex drive all the time and if they don't, their very definition of masculinity is threatened (and heaven forbid they have erectile dysfunction).

It is toxic and tragic. They're not taught how to please us vulva owners. They assume that PIV is the default and if a woman doesn't enjoy it, there is something wrong with her. They don't know that women need their own version of sex (an expanded PIV experience) to stimulate their equivalent erectile tissue/clitoris. They're told women should want to have sex with them whenever they want.

They may even think that women have orgasms the way porn depicts, which is by thrusting with the biggest penis possible, as deep, fast, and hard as they can into the vagina (which is actually how a MAN orgasms). The women in porn are all screaming in ecstasy the minute the guy penetrates so it must be true, right? To which the answer is no. This is a performance. These people are actors. Porn, in most cases, comes from the male perspective and is based on a male fantasy. It is literally designed to get men off as fast as possible.

Thinking porn is reality translates into men trying to please women by being total jackhammers in bed—stick it in fast and go-go-go. The whole time, women are thinking, *Why doesn't this do anything for me?* Add in a fake orgasm, and the whole thing amounts to a total performance disaster for everyone. A fake charade masquerading as sex. Performance-based sex is killing people's sex lives, and it is unfortunately becoming more and more common.

Performance-Based Sex	Pleasure-Based Sex
Needs to be fast	Takes as long as both people want
Is focused on genitals	Considers the whole body an erogenous zone
Includes pressure on one individual to "give" their partner an orgasm	Creates no shame if orgasm doesn't happen
Ends when one partner has an orgasm (usually the male)	Focuses equally on each partner's pleasure and enjoyment
Has a set script that has to happen, usually sequentially	Follows individual needs, desires, and curiosity, and encourages lifelong learning
Can be done wrong and end in failure	Can't be done wrong and can't fail

In a perfect world, everyone would learn the Dr. Kelly Casperson Ideal Version of Sexual Etiquette, which goes like this:

1. Both parties understand: a) the female organ of pleasure is the clitoris, which wraps under the vulva and labia, so they need attention as well, and b) the male organ of pleasure is the penis, and c) lube is good and normal, and should be used liberally.

2. During any sexual encounter, the woman gets to orgasm first WITHOUT a penis in her vagina through oral sex, hands, or toys (unless she prefers and is able to have an orgasm through a penis in her vagina). Once she has an orgasm, THEN the man can put his penis in the vagina (with consent, of course)—if that is his desired way to achieve pleasure when together.

3. Now he can have an orgasm, too, and she can have another one or two as well (but no pressure here at all—just because it is possible for women to have orgasms in quick succession doesn't mean you "should").

4. Everyone is satisfied and happy. They talk about it, and tell each other what worked well and what changes they want to try in the future.

Take a screenshot of those four steps, give it to your partner, put up flyers all over town, post it on your social media, and my job is done here. Problem solved. Everyone's orgasming! (Just kidding—we're just getting started. We still need to talk about so many other physical and mental aspects that contribute to a happy, healthy sex life.)

How Men's Bodies Work

The penis is an amazing organ with three main jobs:

- Pass urine from the bladder to the outside world
- Bring sperm from the testicles/epididymis to the outside world/the female body to continue our species

- Provide pleasure/orgasm for men

The longest part of the penis is called the shaft. At the end of the shaft is the head, or glans, and at the very tip of the head is an opening called the meatus. If a penis is uncircumcised, meaning the foreskin has not been removed, the foreskin covers the glans and can be pulled back or retracted for erection or urination. About 50 percent of penises in the US are circumcised.

The penis is divided into two chambers called the corpora cavernosa (like how the clitoris does that wishbone thing with the chambers we call bulbs). Each chamber contains a multitude of blood vessels and spongy erectile tissue that resembles a loofah. Running along the underside of the penis is the urethra, where urine and sperm exit the body. This is called the corpora spongiosum, the female equivalent of which is the urethra and surrounding spongy erectile tissue called the urethral/clitoral complex.

When sexually stimulated, the brain and nerves signal the corpora cavernosa to relax. This allows blood to rush in, filling up all the spaces in the "loofah." As a result, the penis expands and becomes erect.

Surrounding the corpora cavernosa is a membrane called the tunica albuginea. This traps the blood in the penis by compressing the veins so the erection lasts until the muscles contract again, stopping the inflow of blood and opening up the outflow. This happens either after ejaculation or when the man is no longer aroused. At that point, the blood flows back out.

Ejaculation occurs when stimulation and/or friction makes a man reach peak excitement and release. At that point, the sperm that's been made and stored by the vas deferens and epididymis (small tubes in the testes I like to call sperm college, because that's where the sperm go to mature until they get called upon by the real world) gets pushed into the base of the penis, and the prostate gland and seminal vesicles release secretions called seminal fluid. The two mix to make semen.

Once this happens, there's no stopping an orgasm. The muscles of the penis and pelvic floor contract, forcing semen out the urethra rhythmically. This is called ejaculation. Ejaculation and orgasm are two separate phenomena, but occur simultaneously most times.

After ejaculation, the penis experiences a refractory period. This is when a man's body is "reloading" for another round of sex, so to speak. The refractory period can last hours, or even days as a man ages. Some men have very short refractory periods and can learn to orgasm without ejaculation (but that is quite beyond the scope of this book).

You know what else is great about women's bodies? Our refractory period on average is WAY shorter than men's. They often have to wait to orgasm again, but we can pretty much just keep on having them whenever we want. Yay, us! Short refractory period = multiple orgasms.

Penis Problems

At least, that's USUALLY how it happens. Just like any organ with a job to do, the penis can have some issues. It doesn't always work the way we expect it to.

Sometimes, a man ejaculates sooner than he'd like to. This is referred to as premature ejaculation (PE), and is typically defined as it happening within one minute of penetration (they had to pick a time frame to do research on it). The causes of PE can be biological or psychological, and treatment options include medications, counseling, desensitization, sexual techniques that delay ejaculation, or a combo platter of those. Adjusting expectations and making sure the woman has an orgasm before penetration can also be a great way to manage an orgasmic timing mismatch like PE, so both people are less stressed and more satisfied. Stress and pressure can make PE worse.

And then there's the reason Viagra (Sildenafil)—that "little blue pill"—is sold and has become the most recognized drug in the world: erectile dysfunction (ED). This is when an erection is not firm enough for penetration, or maybe never happens in the first place.

Viagra and all the other drugs in this category work by basically increasing blood flow to the penis and preventing blood flow from leaving, which is helpful for erectile dysfunction caused by these common issues. Of course, not all erection problems are blood flow problems, which is why these meds don't work for everyone.

Before 1998, nearly all erection problems were considered psychogenic—in a man's head. But after Viagra was so successful in helping men with ED, the thinking about its cause was revised to mirror PE's: sometimes it's psychological, sometimes it is physical, and sometimes it is a little of both.

Fun fact: before it became a men's sexual health drug, Sildenafil was actually being studied as a blood pressure medication. When it didn't work very well to lower blood pressure, the researchers asked for the study drug back—but the men didn't WANT to return it, because when they were taking it, something ELSE was going up and staying up. Talk about a blockbuster side effect!

Psychogenic impotence is when there isn't a physical cause for ED. (It is still bizarre to me how something controlled by the brain isn't considered physical—showing our medical establishment's disconnect between brain and body.) It makes the issue seem less real or solvable, but performance anxiety is a real thing. The more anxious, stressed, criticized or "performance-based" a man feels, the worse erectile issues can get. The penis needs a relaxed individual to perform, and a stressed-out body sends signals that this is not an ideal sexy time.

Just a man thinking, *Is it going to work this time or not?* is enough to ruin an erection (the same as when women think, *Why haven't I had an orgasm yet?* or *This is taking too long!* pretty much guarantees she's never going to have one). Once this thought gets stuck in a man's head, ED tends to become a vicious cycle. Even though the pelvis is fully capable of getting an erection, it just doesn't happen. The power of the mind is real, and we can harness it to work for or against us in the bedroom.

Interestingly, studies have shown that 40 percent of the time, a placebo—basically, a sugar pill—gives men an erection. Researchers telling participants, *This is going to make you really hard!* makes their bodies miraculously follow suit. (I'm reminded of a lube I once picked up that had instructions on it: put on the clitoris and rub in a circular motion. Um, that's not the LUBE making you aroused, but okay...) In some female studies, the placebo worked 50 percent of the time for desire. See! Our brain = our biggest sex organ.

Options for psychologically induced ED include anxiety reduction, desensitization, cognitive-behavioral interventions, guided sexual stimulation techniques (often led by a sex therapist), and couples' or relationship counseling. Just taking the pressure off the need for the penis to perform by taking an ED medication can give the penis the boost it needs. Another great option is talking about ways to get pleasure that don't include the penis. The "heterosexual paradigm" of PIV as the only option for sexual activity can be very limiting, so think outside the box (pun intended).

In terms of physical causes, we now know that ED is a canary in the coal mine for heart disease. When blood flow doesn't work well enough to produce an erection, it may be a sign that other arteries in the body are unhealthy. Having diabetes, high cholesterol, metabolic syndrome, poor eating habits, smoking, drinking alcohol, being overweight, sleep deprivation, and not getting enough physical activity all increase a man's risk of having ED as well. I believe if there was a warning on cigarettes that said, *Causes decreased blood flow to the penis and clitoris, leading to eventual penis and clitoris failure*, everyone would quit. Smoking is literally not sexy.

I recently saw a patient with ED who was in his early fifties. He commented, "I guess it's because I'm old, right?" Short answer, no. I see people who are still having fulfilling sex lives well into their nineties. This guy was a longtime (now ex-) smoker with diabetes, high blood pressure, sleep apnea, a weight issue (see below), and was taking multiple medications. I asked if he knew his medical problems were all big contributors to his ED—and he had no idea! See? Men have received no education about how to care for their penises, either.

A note about weight: all bodies are good and are worthy of pleasure. A large range of weights can be healthy. That said, adipose tissue contains a compound called aromatase that converts testosterone to estrogen, which can decrease sex drive and lower available testosterone in both men and women. The good news: any lifestyle change that improves a man's health improves penis health. I told my patient not to give up—that he had potentially forty or more years to enjoy sex. There was no reason to tell his body a toxic lie like you're too old to have reliable erections. I prescribed exercise, a heart-healthy diet, weight loss, and eight hours of sleep a night, and sent him off to get healthier (and harder).

No Penis? No Problem!

Many couples stop having sex because of PE and ED. He was taught that his sexual worth is tied up in his erection and sexual performance, so you can see how he would want to avoid situations where he is reminded of this. Instead of thinking your partner is now unavailable and sex is off the table, ask, *How can we make this work?* That's certainly better than just thinking, *We are not sexual/intimate partners anymore because we couldn't figure out a way around a penis problem.* Because women are socialized in our culture to be the object of desire, we tend to take it super personally when a man can't get or keep an erection. Instead of thinking that's just how his body is working at the moment, we think it's about US—something we did or didn't do, how "good" we are in bed, or that we're not attractive enough, our stomach jiggles too much, or we aren't young enough anymore. NOT TRUE. Erection status does not equal your attractiveness or likability, and it doesn't mean he desires you less. The bigger deal you make out of it, the worse it gets. Penises don't like to be criticized. When in doubt, practice checking in with your penis-owning partner using "I feel" words. For example, "I feel it is about me when you withdraw sexually or lose an erection; can you help me understand it better?"

If Sarah Jessica Parker was playing Carrie Bradshaw in *You Are Not Broken*'s version of *Sex and the City*, she would type on her word processor: *So here's a question for you...can sex exist without a penis?*

The answer is a resounding YES. It's time to start challenging the concept that sex equals PIV and nothing else. Men take pride in pleasing their partner, and non-PIV sex is a great opportunity to do that. It's time to rename foreplay "sex" so everyone can enjoy being sexual no matter what challenges arise. The old way of thinking is like playing music with only two notes. The penis is just one player in the symphony, and you can enjoy a lifetime of sexy fun without making it the star of the show.

So what might this expanded definition of sex and intimacy with your partner look like? (Caution: this is not an exhaustive list.)

- A kissing session, cuddling (clothed or not), holding hands, being emotionally intimate in a way you aren't with anyone else
- Oral sex
- Skin-to-skin contact and touching each other without penetration
- One partner self-cultivating while the other partner watches, or self-cultivating together
- Toys! Experiment with vibrators and dildos—handhelds, ones that provide clitoral suction, and strap-ons. We accept technology in the rest of our lives, so why would sex be the exception?
- Naked or not-naked massage

I've seen relationships literally crumble when couples weren't intimate besides PIV and then it stopped and no one talked about it. Talk early, expand intimacy early. It is preventative maintenance for the future.

Remember, you are not broken, and neither is he. Try having an open, relaxed, and loving conversation. This builds intimacy and opens the doorway to expand what you do together outside the heterosexual paradigm. Even when PE or ED happen, you can both still have fun and enjoy being intimate and sexual together.

So let's hear it for penises and the men we love that they're attached to. Now you know all about how they work (and sometimes, don't). Now you know not to take their function personally, the role you play in pressuring them to perform, and what you make that mean about the human they are attached to. Give them all the love and support you can—they're just trying their hardest.

(Oh how I love puns.)

CHAPTER SIX

Getting All Hormonal

THE PHRASE "YOU'RE SO hormonal!" seems to get thrown at women pretty often, and not in a good way. That must mean hormones are bad, right? NOPE. If we didn't have hormones, we wouldn't be able to propagate the species. In other words, we'd all be dead.

Hormones are not only essential for sex, but for LIFE. We need them to make our entire body function. For instance, there are estrogen receptors in the brain, digestive system, skin and bones, and the heart. They're even in our inner ear (which is why after menopause women tend to get more vertigo)!

And here's another fact you may not know: men and women make the exact same sex hormones, just in different amounts.

MIND-BLOWING, RIGHT?

Contrary to what many of us were taught (or maybe assumed), men aren't the only ones who make testosterone, and women aren't the only ones who make estrogen and progesterone. Both genders make all three, which means our sex drive is being driven by the same chemical messengers. Cool, huh? (Sex drive isn't just from hormones—more on that later—but they do play a part that we need to know about.)

Of course, we make these hormones in different quantities and they are used differently by male and female bodies. Testicles primarily make testosterone, but men make estrogen and progesterone as well. Women primarily produce estrogen and progesterone in the ovaries, but we also produce testosterone in the ovaries and adrenal glands. Our bodies have so many parallels. (Remember, clitoris = penis, ovary = testes. Same idea here.)

Estrogen and Progesterone

Estrogen is the hormone responsible for maintaining female sex characteristics. It helps with women's periods, creates the uterine lining favorable for egg implantation, and keeps the vaginal tissues moist and healthy.

Progesterone is more like a sidekick to estrogen—the Robin to its Batman—with the main job of protecting the uterine lining in the second half of the menstrual cycle to keep the uterus hospitable for implantation and by preventing uterine contractions that would expel an implanted egg. (This is why progesterone levels increase during pregnancy—it's responsible for keeping a baby in the uterus.)

Because progesterone works as a muscle-relaxing hormone, it can also slow the gut and contribute to heartburn and constipation, especially in pregnant women. There is some evidence that progesterone has a calming effect, and may be why we see anxiety go up in the perimenopause years as progesterone drops even before our periods end. Progesterone isn't a huge player in the sexual desire or function scene, but important to know about as an educated human.

Testosterone

Testosterone, also made in the ovaries and, in smaller amounts, in our adrenal glands, is one hormone that contributes to our "get up and go" or zest for life. It's great for creating lean muscle mass, preventing weight gain, and blood and bone health. It is also the hormone responsible for spontaneous sex drive—when the thought of sex pops into your head and you actively go seeking it (more on this in Chapter Eleven: Desire Is So Two-Faced).

This explains why peak desire in premenopausal women commonly happens during ovulation when testosterone and estrogen levels are highest, and why women usually have the most spontaneous sexual desire in their twenties when testosterone levels are at a peak. It also explains why men—who make about ten times more testosterone than women no matter their age—generally have higher levels of spontaneous sex drive throughout their life span (well, that, and they're socialized and permitted to think that way much more than women).

Testosterone goes down after menopause. The role of low testosterone on overall health in women is not well researched at this point, but it is gaining interest as many women choose to use it as an off-label medication after menopause (more on that in Chapter Sixteen: Maybe It's Menopause). Clinical trials suggest that supplementing testosterone enhances cognitive performance, improves musculoskeletal health, and addresses low desire not caused by relationship or other medical issues in postmenopausal women.[17] More research is needed. Volunteers?

Science nerds: testosterone is measured in ng/dl. Normal premenopausal levels are 15–70 ng/dl. Estradiol is measured in pg/ml. Normal premenopausal levels are <50–400 pg/ml. Yes, it fluctuates that much over a menstrual cycle. So let's say at age twenty-eight you have a testosterone level of 40ng/dl, which is equivalent to 400pg/ml. See? Women have a ton of testosterone! It is just one-tenth of what males have, and it has been so gendered in our society that people don't think about us having it (neither do doctors, frankly).

Pop quiz time: does a twenty-five-year-old woman have more estrogen or testosterone in her body?

Answer: it's about equal but depends on the time of the month as estrogen fluctuates so much with the menstrual cycle. Who knew, right?

Hormones and Libido

If our hormone levels get out of whack, does that impact how much we want sex and how often we have it? Sometimes. Hormones are a big deal, but not the whole deal when it comes to desire. Seen in terms of the biopsychosocial model, hormones are the bio part.

Emily Nagoski, in her book *Come as You Are*, explains, "The problem here is that we've been taught to think about sex in terms of behavior, rather than in terms of the biological, psychological and social processes underlying the behavior."

This is called the biopsychosocial model of human sexuality and it takes into account:

Biology: physical health, hormones, medications, lack of appropriate stimulation

Psychology: performance anxiety, limiting thoughts

and beliefs about sexuality, depression, trauma, anxiety, fear, shame, stress, body image

Sociocultural: upbringing, cultural norms, expectations, and how women "should" behave, respond, communicate, and function

Interpersonal: availability of a sexual partner, quality of relationships, lack of emotional intimacy, present and past life stressors, finances, intervals of abstinence, partner support, communication, and expectations.

It acknowledges that sexual response is complex and multifaceted—it's in your body, it's in your brain, it's in your cultural upbringing. It's all of that. Thinking the answer to any issue lies in just one area while ignoring the others generally doesn't lead to a successful outcome. That is why this book includes all of the above, instead of your usual women's magazine fare of "new toys or sex position to have better sex." Those aren't solutions. Understanding your specific biopsychosocial model is.

Journal time: what affects your individual sex life in each category?

1. Your biology:
2. Your psychology:
3. Your social/cultural perspective:
4. Your interpersonal life:

Oral birth control ("the pill") works by preventing the fluctuations of estrogen and progesterone so the ovary doesn't get the signal to release an egg. When oral birth control is processed through the liver, it creates sex-hormone-binding globulin (SHBG). Once the sex hormones become bound up, they're not active or free to be used. While birth control is a fantastic miracle of modern medicine for women—it's allowed us to delay having children while we pursue our dreams and then show our children what is possible!—the downside is it can change the active hormones "seen" by our bodies. This is not a side effect so much as what it is actually designed to do so we don't get pregnant.

As a result of taking the pill, the brain and the vulva sometimes go into low estrogen and testosterone states. This explains why some women on oral birth control come to me complaining of low desire and a dry/painful vulva/vagina. We can't yet predict which women will have these side effects, but the thinking is it is likely a genetic predisposition.

> Men can have low testosterone and still have fine erections, or normal testosterone and still have ED. It's not always correlated. Again, biopsychosocial = we are complicated. Sometimes it would be nicer if life were simpler, right?

Another medication that can block hormones—and as a result, sex drive—is spironolactone. This acne medication blocks acne-causing testosterone. Unfortunately, a lack of testosterone also leads to a lack of sexual desire. It's a total bummer, like *what do you want—clear skin or a sex drive?*

A patient came to me because of decreased sex drive on spironolactone for her acne. It isn't an easy discussion, but luckily in the era of Covid masks and Zoom filters, more women may be comfortable giving up clear skin for the return of spontaneous sex drive. But this is a personal, individualized decision, for sure. Like my good friend and female sex expert Dr. Rachel Rubin says, "When you play with hormones, you get side effects." There can always be consequences to taking hormones as well as blocking them.

If a man complains of low desire, low energy, some weight gain around the middle, decreased muscle mass, and a lack of his normal get-up-and-go—all symptoms of low testosterone—the first thing a doctor will do is check his testosterone level. If it is low, insurance covers periodic injections to get the man's T back into the normal range. No further questions asked. No problem. Not so for women.

There is plenty of research that shows testosterone replacement helps increase sexual desire in women. For example, in a study of thirty-one women in their late thirties (a time when perimenopause can be picking up steam), testosterone therapy resulted in statistically significant improvements in the scores of psychological well-being and sexual self-rating compared with placebo. A mean decrease in the Beck Depression Inventory score approached significance compared to placebo as well. Researchers concluded, "Testosterone therapy improves well-being, mood, and sexual function in premenopausal women with low libido and low testosterone. As a substantial number of women experience diminished sexual interest and well-being during their late reproductive years, further research is warranted to evaluate the benefits and safety of longer-term intervention."[18]

Another study looking at perimenopausal women in their forties found that transdermal testosterone therapy improved well-being, mood, and sexual function.[19] Still more research showed that satisfying sexual events were greater when taking testosterone than a placebo for SSRI-related (antidepressant) female sexual dysfunction (2.3 events versus 0.1 events a month).[20] Adjacently, vaginal estrogen therapy has also been found to positively affect sexual function in that it improves arousal, lubrication, and sexual comfort.

So why don't we treat women suffering decreased desire caused by low testosterone by giving them testosterone replacement? For starters, by thinking of testosterone as the "male hormone," we demonstrate an inherent bias against women needing it. Yet we know postmenopausal women have low testosterone, just like they have low estrogen and progesterone. It would go a long way to start thinking of testosterone as a hormone BODIES—not just male bodies—have, especially when trying to help women with their quality of life in regards to their sexuality. Another barrier: even though the above data shows that low testosterone levels are closely correlated with decreased coital frequency and loss of desire, other studies say there's no correlation at all. And so as of now, that means the medical recommendation remains that testosterone levels should not be used to "check or test" for female sexual dysfunction. Until things change, you may need to advocate at your doctor's office if you think testosterone sounds right for you to try. There are new guidelines for dosing testosterone for postmenopausal low desire they can access.[21]

Keep in mind, testosterone is not safe for a pregnancy so it is not recommended in premenopausal women. In addition, premenopausal women are assumed to have normal hormones so other reasons for low desire should be investigated first. That said, perimenopause can start affecting hormones much earlier than many people think, years before your periods stop. Another caveat: there are always side effects to taking any medication, and there are also things you can do to enhance sexual desire without hormone therapy (more on that later).

Keeping Hormones Healthy

A healthy body promotes healthy hormones. You can enhance your health by getting adequate amounts of sleep; eating earth-based foods that are not factory created or processed; avoiding alcohol (a known hormone disrupter), caffeine, and smoking (tobacco, cannabis, or anything else); moving your body frequently; reducing stress; and yes, having more sex, including oral sex and self-cultivation (don't just assume PIV; we are better than that now). Some studies even show that sexually active women have later onset of menopause. The theory is that the body thinks reproduction could still be possible (even if we protect against it) and keeps the brain telling the ovaries to keep on the job.[22]

Also, there is no such thing as hormone balance. This is a marketing gimmick used by someone trying to sell you something. If hormones were "balanced," no monthly fluctuations would happen, periods would stop, and pregnancies wouldn't occur. Also, postmenopause, there is no balance, unless you consider "all hormones low" to be "balanced."

If there is anything that needs to be balanced, I would say it is our stress levels. Increased cortisol—the stress hormone—and living a stressful lifestyle can decrease our sex hormones. Increased cortisol = increased sympathetic nervous system activity, which puts us "on alert." Focusing on our parasympathetic nervous system makes us more relaxed and calmer in the present moment, which results in more great sex becoming available to us. As a surgeon I think I spent fifteen years in sympathetic drive. I now actively work on my parasympathetic nervous system to counter years of being "off balance" cortisol- and stress-wise.

I'm making progress, which doesn't come by hoping or wishing. It is work, but work that restores balance in life. So if a lackluster sex life turns out to be your wake-up call to reevaluate your health, stress, busyness, and communication skills, please consider it to be a transformational and life-changing gift.

I'll leave you with one more thought here: hormones are not dirty words. They are not bad, or bad for you (more on this later when I talk about what else is coming—menopause!). Hormones are essential for a happy sex life, and a healthy life in general, so make sure yours are doing their very important jobs efficiently.

CHAPTER SEVEN

The Chemistry of Pleasure

JUST LIKE HORMONES, neurotransmitters—chemicals made in the brain—can impact how much or little we want to have sex. The two main neurotransmitters of pleasure are dopamine and serotonin. But while dopamine increases desire, serotonin often puts the brakes on it.

Say what? How can two chemicals both give us pleasure, but one makes us WANT to have sex and the other says, NAH, NOT TONIGHT?

Dopamine is responsible for our seeking behavior. Seeking behavior = desire for something. It acts as a reward by giving us a total rush. Sex, sugar, and drugs all hit our dopamine receptors, but it is not only the actual substance that rewards us—it is also the amazing high that comes from seeking those things out.

You may be asking yourself: if dopamine is the neurotransmitter of desire, why don't we just give people drugs that stimulate dopamine? The answer is, these kinds of drugs are given to Parkinson's patients who have movement problems stemming from decreased dopamine in a specific part of their brain—and sometimes the side effects of taking them include hypersexuality; compulsive eating, gambling, and shopping; and in rare cases, criminal behavior. So while we may THINK what we want is increased desire, when we literally increase it, we get behaviors that don't work well for the life we want to live. Dopamine drugs show us we can't just "pick and choose" what effects we want, or at least not yet.

On the other hand, the pleasure serotonin brings is more about contentment than exhilaration. It makes us feel satisfied, happy, and mellow. That doesn't exactly give us any motivation to seek out sex...or anything.

This is why antidepressants in the most commonly prescribed selective serotonin reuptake inhibitor (SSRI) category—meaning they keep more serotonin around the brain—are known to lift depression but decrease sex drive and the ability to orgasm. To avoid this kind of sexual dysfunction, some people choose antidepressants associated with less decrease in sexual function such as bupropion, mirtazapine, vortioxetine, vilazodone, or even the serotonin and norepinephrine reuptake inhibitors (SNRI) duloxetine and desvenlafaxine. Ask your doctor before changing any meds on your own.

Here are some things that impact dopamine and serotonin levels in the body:

- Cortisol dampens dopamine—stress is clearly not good for seeking out sex. I explain a majority of women's low desire for sex with this singular fact.
- Iron deficiency (anemia) makes it harder for the body to create and process dopamine or serotonin as effectively, putting a damper on both mood and the ability to get IN the mood.

- Magnesium deficiency may contribute to decreased dopamine levels and an increased risk of depression. If you don't get enough magnesium in your diet, especially in the peri- and menopausal age groups, a supplement can be considered.
- Vitamin D exerts protective and regulatory effects on the brain dopamine system.
- Testosterone increases dopamine release, adding to spontaneous sexual desire. It has also been shown to potentially assist in serotonin uptake in the brain, enhancing mood.
- Exercise, a healthy diet, and proper sleep can also contribute to increased dopamine and serotonin release in the brain.
- Anticipating sex (being around sexual stimuli) and orgasm itself releases dopamine. Unsatisfying sex (no pleasure, no orgasm) breaks the reward pathway in the brain = the less you enjoy sex the less you seek it out.

Fun fact: music also increases dopamine by stimulating the same areas in the brain as sex and drugs. Yup, what you've always suspected is true—music is sexy. It also increases our ratings of the attractiveness of others while listening to music.

So can we hijack this knowledge to increase sexual desire? YES! We can prime the brain with one stimulating thing and use it to get stimulated about something else. Going super neuroscience here, this is called cross-modal transfer of arousal. In one study, researchers asked heterosexual college students to listen to music, look at pictures of the opposite sex, and then rank their attractiveness. Results showed that "women, but not men, gave significantly higher ratings of facial attractiveness and dating desirability after having listened to music than in the silent control condition. High-arousing, complex music yielded the largest effects, suggesting that music may affect human courtship behavior through induced arousal."[23]

In another, they put people on roller coasters then asked them to rate the attractiveness of some "average" photographs of the opposite gender (again, this was heterosexual research). The results were that "people reported higher degrees of sexual attractiveness and dating desirability towards a photograph of an opposite-sex individual of average attractiveness after exiting the ride, in comparison to people tested before entering the ride."[24]

So, what does this tell us? Exercise, music, roller coasters, whatever gets your brain thrilled will increase your desire. GET EXCITED! It also explains why doing novel, fun things with your significant other can increase your desire for them.

One woman told my ob-gyn friend how offended she was when her doctor told her to "date" her husband. I don't find this is offensive at all. It simply uses human psychology to harness the power of our dopamine attractiveness-seeking pathways. If we don't spend time with our significant others, have fun, explore the world, and do something other than the daily serious business of being adults, we shouldn't be surprised when our drive goes down.

So there it is again—you are not broken. You just need a proverbial roller coaster to put more "seeking" into your life. I know you can't go to an amusement park every Friday night, but research has also shown that listening to comedy or a "thriller" type story also has the same effect. Whatever works for you, do that!

The last neurotransmitter you need for your sex education is oxytocin. It is a bonding (or love/cuddle molecule) released with breastfeeding and orgasm. It is why you may feel sleepy and relaxed after sex. Oxytocin also has pain-relieving properties, which is why people say sex is good at relieving menstrual cramps and headaches, and decreasing symptoms of the common cold. Studies are mixed as to whether giving people oxytocin improves their sex lives.

Anyone want to quit their day job and become a sex researcher yet?

CHAPTER EIGHT

Own Your Orgasm

FUN FACT: THE thinking brain, called the prefrontal cortex, literally shuts down during orgasm. You can't do math, make a grocery list, or plan your summer vacation. There is no higher cognitive function, just pleasure. Sounds nice, huh?

While there is a clear reason for male orgasm beyond just feeling good (and that is to push sperm out of the body), people argue that there is no good reason for a female orgasm. Evolution didn't take a logic class and I love her for that, but we are left guessing. During the Victorian era, it was believed men and women had to simultaneously orgasm for pregnancy to happen—that the muscular contractions working together were necessary for the sperm to fertilize an egg. However, there is no evidence that orgasm has a role to play in making a woman pregnant.[25] Since then women's orgasm has fallen to the wayside. It is considered an unnecessary, expendable homologue without any "use."

I dissent, your honor. This view devalues the role of women's pleasure compared to men. Women's pleasure makes our bodies open up, literally and figuratively. With arousal, our vagina widens and lengthens and we want to draw in, embrace, have someone be close to us (when we aren't self-cultivating, that is). Our orgasm equipment, the literal buttons, are out front and center (although with how much our names of the body parts and images are considered "dirty" on social media, I would say for most women it is hidden in plain sight—it's there but we aren't aware, thus, this book).

Some research suggests orgasms persist because they actually have a very important function—they feel amazing, so they encourage women to have sex (no sex = no humans). One theory states women have orgasms because men have them—again the clitoris and penis are the same embryological structure—kind of like how male nipples will never go away because they are so important to the female. Another theory is that if a male partner gives his partner orgasms (a.k.a., he cares enough), he is a good choice for having children with and keeping around longer. Many mammals need sex to ovulate. This is not true in humans, but perhaps we used to need to as well? History and Mother Nature aren't talking, so of course this is all speculation.

Female orgasms last longer than men's and can occur rapidly in succession. That is a lot of energy for something with "no function." Sex that feels good is important in a social, pair-bonded species. It helps partners stay connected. We have evolved to appreciate the pleasure of staring at ocean waves, fires, and music, so why is pleasure with sex ever questioned as not being beneficial?

Here are some things we do know, other than just how good orgasms feel. In both sexes they:

- Help you feel closer to your partner (by releasing oxytocin, the social bonding hormone)

- Decrease stress and anxiety
- Promote relaxation (some researcher compared an orgasm to a dose of Valium)
- Stimulate sleep and reduce insomnia
- Help pass kidney stones. (No, really! Orgasm has been shown to facilitate passing distal ureteral stones. So do roller coaster rides. The urologist in me digresses...)
- Boost the immune system by releasing leukocytes and natural killer cells[26]
- Decrease pain (including the discomfort of menstrual cramps in women)
- Promote neuron growth in the hippocampus (important for memory and learning), as shown in both animal and human studies

All great reasons for having more orgasms, right? But wait, there's more.

Want to live as long as possible? Research shows that men who have two or more orgasms a week die at half the rate of those who orgasm less than once a month.[27] We don't have great orgasm/longevity data in women, but in a twenty-five-year longitudinal study looking at predictors of longevity, the strongest three factors for the women were: health satisfaction, past enjoyment of intercourse, and their rating of their physical function.[28]

I'm not trying to "should" you, but I do want you to know that orgasms are a healthy thing. Also, I need to counter all the people and teachings that told you sex is bad. Our bodies reward us with such awesome side effects because evolution wants us to have sex. Yes, pleasure is reason enough to have an orgasm, but boosting our well-being, cardiac health, and lifespan are nothing to sneeze at, either.

Time for another pop quiz! Who has the most orgasms?

A. Women with women
B. Men with men
C. Men with women
D. Women with men

The Orgasm Gap

When it comes to who has the most—and most reliable—orgasms, heterosexual men are the clear winner, followed closely by gay men. Lesbians are in third place, and trailing in dead last are heterosexual women. In a large sample of fifty-two thousand Americans, data shows that "Heterosexual men were most likely to say they usually or always orgasmed when sexually intimate (95 percent), followed by gay men (89 percent), bisexual men (88 percent), lesbian women (86 percent), bisexual women (66 percent), and heterosexual women (65 percent)."[29]

Why does such a wide orgasm gap exist? I think the common belief that sex ends when the man orgasms and ejaculates, and that PIV sex is the be all and end all in hetero sex (which doesn't make most women orgasm) are the most likely culprits. Experts call this the "phallocentric imperative," which I kind of love.[30] So many people think just putting things in the vagina is what's supposed to get women there. Same-sex female couples probably have an easier time with orgasm because they don't have that PIV paradigm to worry about.

You literally put a penis in the room and her orgasms go down. We know this because we have data on bisexual women's orgasm frequency when partnered with men and women. Nothing like a randomized control study, where women went (on average) from orgasming 64 percent of the time when with another woman to 7 percent when partnered with a man.[31]

Maher, Mintz, and Akers believe orgasmic inequality exists due to:

1. Cultural overvaluing of intercourse and men's sexual pleasure (while at the same time undervaluing women's sexual pleasure and clitoral stimulation).
2. Women's lack of entitlement to sexual pleasure. They say "the bar is low—'absence of pain and degradation'—rather than as the presence of pleasure and orgasm."
   a. going in with expectations to not orgasm
   b. valuing partner's orgasm more than their own
   c. not knowing that orgasms come from clitoral stimulation and faking them to protect partner's ego
3. Cognitive distractions during sexual encounters—appearance focused, performance anxiety, and I would add not being mentally turned on or "into it."

Their tips for closing the orgasm gap include:

- normalize female orgasms as equal.
- empower women to figure out the stimulation they need and transfer to partnered sex.
- rewrite the script from foreplay → intercourse → male ejaculation to turn-taking scripts such as she comes first, then he comes with PIV (or preferred); foreplay, he comes, she comes with vibrator; and/or intercourse with clitoral stimulation.

We have to own our sexuality, find out what works for us, and teach our partners what that is. It is not true that men should just know what they're doing. We're not Toyotas (all built the same) and we don't come with an owner's manual. And if we don't know how to tap into our body for pleasure, we can't communicate about it with our partner.

Cultivating Your Orgasm

Orgasms need to be cultivated and discovered. They don't exist in our normal high-stress, multitasking world. You have to be in your body and in the moment. Like any physical activity, the more you master it, the easier, better, and more fluid it becomes.

And speaking of physical activity...women with weak pelvic floors have more difficulty achieving orgasm, so start doing your Kegels. Doing pelvic floor exercises has been shown to increase and enhance orgasmic abilities. In fact, a 2021 study showed that twelve weeks of daily lifting of the pelvic floor for at least six seconds was enough to decrease sexual dysfunction.[32] Pelvic-floor-trained physical therapists are a godsend. Check out hermanwallace.com to find one near you.

Compared to women who orgasmed less frequently, women who orgasmed more frequently were more likely to: receive more oral sex, have longer duration of the last sexual episode, be more satisfied with their relationship, ask for what they want in bed, praise their partner for something they did in bed, call/email to tease about doing something sexual, wear sexy lingerie, try new sexual positions and anal stimulation, act out fantasies, incorporate sexy talk, and express love during sex. Women were more likely to orgasm if their last sexual encounter included deep kissing, manual genital stimulation, and/or oral sex in addition to vaginal intercourse."[33]

A Finnish study looked at what made some women more successful with orgasms than others. It concluded that, "The keys to their more frequent orgasms lay in mental and relationship factors.

These factors and capacities included orgasm importance, sexual desire, sexual self-esteem, and openness of sexual communication with partners. In addition, positive determinants were the ability to concentrate, mutual sexual initiations, and partner's good sexual techniques. A relationship that felt good and worked well emotionally, and where sex was approached openly and appreciatively, promoted orgasms."[34]

Arousal needs to happen in the brain as much or more than the pelvis. We aren't light switches. Figuring out how to get your brain into a sexy context is a very useful skill when you want to go from daytime boss/mom/cortisol sympathetic nervous system to Pleasantville.

Remember, pleasure is the overall goal. Orgasm is a sign of pleasure, but if you make the orgasm the goal, you have just created performative, goal-oriented sex, which ironically makes us less likely to orgasm. Many sexperts think that the orgasm shouldn't be the "end all" for people, and I want you to hear and feel that side of things, too.

If you need a little more help figuring out how to make yourself feel good and/or orgasm, two great online resources are omgyes.com and dodsonandross.com. (Betty Dodson, famed sexologist and driving force behind dodsonandross.com, believes you must become connected to yourself by masturbation in order to bring this knowledge to partnered sex.) Both offer a variety of illuminating techniques, education, and information that will help you get where you want to go. Remember, our bodies were built for pleasure, and you have everything you need to enjoy yours.

Self-Cultivation for the Win

While the same Finnish study I referenced above didn't find self-cultivation helped women orgasm better with their partner, other research does support this. Specifically, data has been shown that masturbation practice can assist less experienced women in reaching orgasm during partnered sex.

But you can't communicate what works for you to your partner if you haven't figured out the instruction manual first, so find out what you like on your own. There are so many things you can learn that way, such as:

- What do you like?
- What makes you come fast or hard?
- What makes you come slow, taking a long, relaxing, rhythmic time?
- What's uncomfortable?
- What's a hard stop, absolute no?
- What's an absolute must?

Practice mindfulness when self-cultivating. When touching your clitoris, BE your clitoris. Pretend your breath is coming from your pelvis as you draw it in and out. If your mind wanders, bring your breath back into your pelvis and practice staying there. Try rubbing your clitoris a little more softly, in a circular motion, or higher up on the glans and shaft. Go back to massaging the labia. Change positions if you need to. Get curious about what feels good and do more of that!

Vibrators and erotica are also long-standing recommendations to enhance physical and psychological sexual stimulation. Female-friendly options for both exist and they can be pretty great. The new kids on the block are clitoral stimulators best described as giving wavelike pulses to the clitoris. I call them "the finishers" because they are great for climaxing with solid consistency. Some women say they almost work *too* well, and don't like them because it ends too fast and feels too automatic and "light switch-y." Other women love them, and use them after a nice romp or as a "companion" when traveling.

Experimenting with a vibrator doesn't mean you're replacing your partner, and I'm not only suggesting you use one by yourself. Many couples who care about women's orgasmic equality use them together. (And in case you're worried about it, there is no data showing that vibrators are addictive.)

Are you already thinking, *Nah, that's not for me*? Try thinking of it this way instead: if you go to a restaurant and someone always orders you chicken, there's no way to know what else you might like on the menu. If you have been having sex "this way" your whole life you literally have no idea what else is on the menu unless you explore. Own your body and its ability to feel pleasure. Do this for no one else but you.

Sexual agency—knowing what you want and don't want—is the common denominator of sexually satisfied women. For those of you who feel like you need it, here is some permission to try new things. Some pointers to keep in mind while you're learning:

- Respect where you are without shame. We all started from not knowing and no one is grading you
- Know that learning requires repetition and making mistakes
- Practice with no agenda other than pleasure
- Bored? Then you are not learning! No one desires boring sex. If you want to "fix" your desire, you must seek something that isn't boring.

Empowering Sexual Confidence

Gather your courage and start building your self-confidence. Your regular, garden-variety confidence is based on what you did in the past—like *I have confidence I can swim a lap in the pool because I've done that a million times before.* But SELF-confidence comes from having your own back while learning to swim. See the difference? You don't need evidence to have self-confidence—it is ALWAYS available. Start by telling yourself *I believe in me unconditionally and it is okay to be curious. I am working to make my sexuality my own. I choose to prioritize my pleasure.* Try and fail, rinse and repeat, and see where that takes you.

There is a reason women call discovering themselves sexually an "awakening." Once you see sexuality is possible, an important part of your personal growth, and a vital part of owning a human body, you will be unstoppable. Many experts believe sexually confident women are also unstoppable at work (and anywhere else she takes these tools of self-agency, self-confidence, curiosity, and pleasure). This kind of growth overflows into all aspects of your life.

There is an agency, life force, and conviction that comes from having your own back and ownership over your own life as an equal to others around you. Start experiencing living life for YOU, not for someone else or waiting for x, y, and z to be perfect. Vow to live perfectly imperfect—without "shoulding" yourself anymore—because the journey is the whole point.

And most of all, have fun. You are the creator of your pleasure, and orgasmic equality is worth pursuing.

CHAPTER NINE

Communication Is Lubrication

ONCE UPON A time there was a woman who absolutely LOVED having her nipples kissed, so she always kissed her partner's nipples during sex and figured he'd get the hint. Instead, he started to kiss her nipples less and less frequently until he almost never did it anymore. Exasperated, she finally said, "It really turns me on when you kiss my nipples, so I tried to convey that by kissing YOURS. What's the deal?" He told her he'd be happy to kiss her nipples—but that he HATED having it done to him, and he'd tried to show her that by NOT kissing hers.

Or how about this one? A couple went to therapy because they were bored and had "no desire" for sex. But when the therapist talked to each partner individually and asked what they thought might turn them on, both mentioned kink. They'd never talked about it to each other for fear of being judged. Once they had the conversation, they started exploring new things, going to kink conventions together, and were thrilled with their sex life.

> Two great apps that take the pressure off of revealing what you'd like to try with your partner are quiv.re and mojoupgrade.com. These free quizzes allow each partner to swipe right and left on all sorts of sexual situations, and then only show the two of you the ones you both matched on—no embarrassment necessary!

What can we learn from them? If there's any place we could all use a good lesson in communication skills, it's in partnered sex. You're literally naked with another human and nobody tells you how to talk to each other about it. Instead, we ASSUME we know what our partners (and people in general) are thinking and get ourselves into all kinds of trouble.

Our assumptions often come from the "manuals" we make in our minds that outline how everyone is supposed to act. For instance, your partner might have a manual for you that you should have sex with him three times a week. If you don't, he might make it mean that you have low desire or aren't attracted to him anymore. None of that is true. You're just not living his manual. Likely he never shared his manual with you and you have never read it, yet here you are feeling bad and there he is feeling rejected.

Or maybe you have a manual for your partner that he shouldn't ask for sex when you are stressed because that's a turnoff for you, he only enjoys sex in the missionary position, or he should snuggle you whenever you want without you having to tell him. Then when he doesn't read your mind by knowing you're in the mood to cuddle, you make it mean that you're unlovable and he is annoying and boring. That's not what's really happening, so what if you just told him what's up in your head instead? Let him "read" your manual by sharing it with him.

You: Hey, when you want to watch a sporting event instead of snuggling with me, I feel unlovable.

Him: The Super Bowl is exciting, but of course I love you too! I wasn't even thinking about cuddling. Thanks for telling me how you feel. Just ask me for a cuddle next time, my love.

The moral of the story here is, no one is a mind reader. You have to actually TALK to each other. *Ugh,* you might be thinking. *That sounds so awkward.* Yup, it probably will be awkward, at least at first. So what? Do it anyway. And repeat and repeat. Repetition is the key to adult learning. Don't worry, we can do hard things. The vulnerability revealed in learning how to communicate about difficult things is where intimacy is found.

Here are some tips to get you started.

- **Timing matters.** Be dressed and give a heads-up. Say something like, "Hey, tomorrow after dinner, I really want to talk about our sex life," so it's not a surprise. Don't try to have a conversation when you're naked in bed after a failed sexual event!
- **Tone matters, too. Use "I" and "we" statements.** I have been learning about orgasm inequality. I have been reading about female sexual response. We can give each other even more pleasure if we talk about what turns us on. "You" sounds judgmental and puts your partner on the defensive.
- **Formulate "what" and "how" questions.** What is the biggest challenge here? How can I help make this better for us? What brought us to this place? How can we solve this problem? "Why" sounds like an accusation and puts us on the defensive, but open-ended questions open up the brain to try to help and solve problems.

- **Say "Tell me everything!"** People love this. Who doesn't want to hear that?!? Then listen without judgment. People can tell when you are listening and when you are trying to think of how to respond. Drop the responding part—just hear the words. Learning how to listen = superpower.

- **Practice mirroring.** Match your partner's eye contact, energy, volume, and pace of talking as a way to increase trust. Even monkeys do this, meaning it is hardwired into us. One study even found that men rated women who mimicked them more positively as potential mates.[35]

- **Ditch the agenda.** Bring only curiosity and fascination into your conversation. View this as a learning experiment. See where you get and realize this isn't just a onetime conversation.

- **Expect differences.** You're not living with your twin, and it can be fascinating and shocking to realize other people think differently than us. If you go into this believing your partner thinks exactly the same way you do, you're wrong. (Man, oh man, why do I have to keep relearning this over and over and over again in my life?)

- **Ask questions and share answers.** Discuss how you learned about sex and how it was talked about in your family. Define what sex means to you both—is it PIV or naked cuddles or everything in between? (Hint: until you understand what sex means to you and what you want to get out of it, you can't possibly know what it means to somebody else.) Challenge your limiting beliefs.

- **Hear them out.** Practice active listening skills. (Again, if you're just thinking about what you want to say next, you're not listening.) Try to understand their manuals—for you, for women, for sex. Hear their responses without making things mean anything other than what they are saying. Give your partner ample space to communicate and credit for trying. Ask clarifying questions.

- **Compromise but beware of "mismatched shoes."** In *Never Split the Difference* by former FBI terrorist negotiator Chris Voss, he uses the example of a woman wanting her husband to wear black shoes and the man wanting to wear brown, so he wears one of each—and no one ends up happy. Come up with mutually agreeable solutions instead. And remember that no means no. Consent is always sexy. Coercion is not.

- **Recognize the problem is the unsolved issue, not your partner.** Voss also reminds us that the person we are talking with is never the problem. Viewing our partner as part of the solution opens up the world instead of shutting it down. See? Taking tips from a hostage negotiator can be good for your sex life!

- **Keep at it.** Every problem—ED, pregnancy, menopause, life stressors, a health scare—could be the end of your sex life if you don't keep communicating. Learn to say things like, "I'm breastfeeding, so it's not pleasurable to have my breasts touched at the moment. Right now my body needs to be touched in a different way. I still love you 100 percent; let's try to figure this out together."

- **Male partners don't know anything else.** He was taught that sex = PIV. That's working out pretty great for him, right? So it may come as a big surprise that PIV doesn't work for most women. And that your decreased interest in sex isn't that you don't enjoy it as much as he does, but that you actually do more work around the house and are tired all the time. You have the data and knowledge on your side now. He still needs to learn what "good sex" is for you and what you need to take off the brakes and press the accelerator on your desire and orgasm. Teach him!

Like I've said before, sex is the only thing everyone is supposed to be an expert at, but nobody got any training. We don't want to sound dumb so we don't ask questions. But how do you get to be an expert? By learning, practicing, and making changes based on feedback.

And feedback means TALKING. If you never get any feedback, you could easily be practicing the wrong things. Like kissing the nipples, or not kissing the nipples. By staying bored because you're scared to mention your interest in kink or just a change in pace, positions, or routine. Sexually satisfied couples are the ones who discuss sex!

Pay close attention to "What am I making this mean?" Never assume you know someone's intent. Our brains are meaning-making machines but that doesn't mean they are accurate—like, ever. Listen, repeat back, and ask for clarification. Bonus points, your partner will feel heard.

Of course, you can't expect that after a single talk, your partner will go buy you an incredible vibrator, read *She Comes First* cover to cover, and you'll magically start having sex and multiple mind-blowing orgasms every day. (I mean, we can dream, but that's just not realistic.) I encourage you to practice a LIFETIME of communication. Learning how to communicate our needs in a relationship is key to a good sex life. My biggest piece of advice here is: always come from love. When you don't know what to do or say, ask, *What would love do in this situation*? Work toward that "good enough" long-term, sustainable sexuality. Don't strive for a performance you saw once in a movie.

Allow yourself to be vulnerable. Brené Brown, who researches courage, vulnerability, shame, and empathy, challenges us to "show up and be seen when we can't control the outcome." Remember communication is where intimacy lies precisely because of the uncertainty, risk, and emotional exposure we share with each other.

If you're thinking, *It should be easy because the rest of our relationship is so good*, that is simply not true. Even the best couples struggle with intimacy. Put in the effort—nothing will ever be more worth it.

Good sex doesn't exist in a vacuum. Research has repeatedly shown that a satisfying, active sex life depends on the strength of the relationship and availability of the partner. If the relationship is stressed or strained, it is highly likely that sex is infrequent and strained as a result.

Renowned couples therapist Dr. John Gottman created a model called the Four Horsemen of the Apocalypse. It offers a good reminder of behaviors that are toxic to relationships.

1. Criticism—need I explain this one?
2. Contempt—attacking the sense of self with an intent to insult or abuse. Gottman's research shows this is the single greatest predictor of divorce.
3. Defensiveness—victimizing oneself to ward off a perceived attack or reverse the blame.
4. Stonewalling—withdrawal to avoid conflict and convey disapproval, distance, and separation.

Learn more about the four horsemen and their antidotes at gottman.com.

PART THREE

Is It *Actually* Low Desire— or Something Else Entirely?

CHAPTER TEN

It Might Not Even Be a "You" Problem

MASTERS AND JOHNSON were the first contemporary team to try to categorize exactly what was happening in the human body during sex. Their research was observational, based on watching people have sex in a lab. This led to the development of a four-stage, linear sexual response cycle: Excitement, Plateau, Orgasm, and Resolution. They didn't even consider desire a necessary component of sex. (Although if you volunteer to have sex in front of researchers in a lab in the 1950s, I guess your desire can be pretty much assumed.)

In 1974, Helen Singer Kaplan—a science-based sex therapist who founded the first clinic to treat sexual disorders—consolidated the Masters and Johnson model into three phases. She combined the Excitement and Plateau stages (because most people were like,

Plateau? What's that?), eliminated Resolution as she saw it more as a lack of sexual response than a phase itself, and then added a new stage before excitement—DESIRE. Called Kaplan's Triphasic Model of Sexual Response, it looks like this: Desire, Excitement, Orgasm.

Ah! Now we're getting somewhere! you might be thinking. Unfortunately, her model is simple but not inclusive of all experiences. Desire doesn't always come first for women. Desire is not always separate from arousal. Orgasm doesn't always come last—it could come in the middle, or not at all. Women can desire sex even after they have an orgasm.

Not to mention, women have so many reasons for having sex other than desire. In research published in their book *Why Women Have Sex*, Cindy Mesters and David Buss identified 237 distinct sexual motivations. Two hundred and thirty-seven! They broke these into four quadrants: Physical (example: to burn calories), goal-based (example: to have a baby), emotional (example: to feel connected), and insecurity-based (example: for attention). Go listen to Episode 20 of my podcast *You Are Not Broken* to hear me read the entire list—it's like a spoken-word poetry jam.

Both Masters and Johnson and Kaplan are often criticized for being male-centric, explaining men's experiences more accurately than women's and focusing on the body's experience over the psychological, emotional, and relationship contexts. Good thing, then, that Rosemary Basson came along and realized that while MALE sexual response generally starts with sexual desire, leads to arousal, and ends in orgasm, the process is not nearly as linear in females. OF COURSE desire can come before or after arousal. OF COURSE orgasm isn't a given. OF COURSE relationship satisfaction and availability of a willing partner are big contributors to whether women even engage in sex or not. And the ultimate biggie: spontaneous sex drive is not usually why women have sex.

Many times women seek emotional intimacy, which then leads to pursuing sexual intimacy, which results in arousal and desire. There is actually a name for this: demisexual, meaning someone who feels sexual attraction to a person only once they've emotionally bonded with them. Totally normal.

Rosemary Basson's theory was a great step forward. Too bad most people don't know about it. Maybe that's why many women still believe the way we desire sex should mirror the male experience, and somehow sex should be natural and easy. We compare and despair, thinking everyone besides us is happy and having great sex. (To which I say, *Knock it off!* Whether they are or aren't is none of your business anyway.)

I want you to know that there are SO many factors that can contribute to less-than-desirable desire levels. Besides, there isn't even a set definition for low libido. One might be "lower than you want," but I think what we have been told we should want is based on male function and Hollywood fantasy, so I don't like that definition either. And if we haven't defined it, how can we be broken by it?

While hypoactive sexual desire disorder (HSDD) is a valid, legitimate diagnosis with FDA-approved medications to treat it, low desire is not always—or even usually—caused by a neurochemical imbalance. (More on HSDD later.) Sometimes it is the world we live in and how we function/exist in said world that causes low desire. The top culprits are societal and psychological pressures. Biological and/or physical can pile on top of that, too. It might even be a combo platter of all of the above.

If you're experiencing lower desire than you'd like, which biopsychosocial factors do you think might be contributing to it? Is there anything you can do to mitigate those factors? Who can you enlist to help you?

Desire Mismatch

Another thing many women experience and mistakenly label as "low desire" is known as sexual desire discrepancy (SDD)—when partners in a relationship want different levels of sexual activity. Maybe there are some unicorn couples out there with the exact same desire level, but that isn't the default. People have different desires about a lot of things: how often the house should be cleaned, when and where to take a vacation, if it's appropriate to have pizza and no vegetables for dinner. Sex is just another example of this that we need to normalize.

SDD is extremely common. There is absolutely nothing wrong with you because you want sex more or less frequently than someone else. It is not the low-desire person's job to be fixed to rise to the level of the high-desire person's needs and wants. The only problem comes when you don't talk about it. That's where shame, assumptions, and avoidance can creep in.

For example, let's say the higher desire person keeps hounding the lower desire person because they think, *My partner says yes one out of every seven times, so I have to ask for sex every day to get it once a week.* Then the lower-desire partner starts to feel badgered and like they say no all the time (which they do), and sex becomes a chore. That leads to avoidance, going to bed at different times to avoid sex, and not touching at all because it may lead to sex. Ugh. No one ends up happy in this scenario!

The European Society for Sexual Medicine suggests the following steps for couples who are distressed by SDD:

- Normalize and depathologize variation in sexual desire in a paired romantic relationship
- Educate about the natural course of sexual desire: that spontaneous desire decreases with an increase in the length of relationships and that spontaneous and responsive desire are

both common and normal
- Emphasize the age-related and relative nature of SDD
- Challenge the myth of spontaneous sexual desire as the default and preferred
- Promote open sexual communication
- Assist in developing joint sexual scripts that are mutually satisfying in addition to the search for personal sexual needs
- Deal with relationship issues and unmet relationship needs
- Stimulate self-differentiation, defined as the ability to relate to your partner without losing one's healthy sense of self, and not losing connection to your own needs while still having a deep connection to your partner, whose views may differ from yours[36]

In other words, SDD is NORMAL, and the best thing to do is talk about it with your partner so you're both on the same page. No, that does not mean you have to adjust your desire to match theirs. It is not your job to fulfill your partner's every need or vice versa. The "right amount" is what is right for the relationship. It may be a middle ground for both.

If your partner wants to have sex three times a week and you don't, that's okay. Your sex drive is not wrong and the other person's is not right. It's not you versus what society says is normal. You are not competing with anybody else. There should be no comparison—this is about you living your best life with your partner.

People often ask me what is "normal." I don't tell them. Averages are just that—and within two standard deviations of the average is still considered normal—so that is a huge range of normal. Specifying a particular number of times a week makes people think quantity is more important than quality and sex becomes a to-do list item, just like eating five to eight fruits and vegetables, doing thirty to fifty minutes of exercise, and getting eight hours of sleep a day. Boom, way to make it a checklist chore. So no, don't do that to yourselves. That said, Barry McCarthy believes sexual desire is facilitated by a "rhythm of regular sexual experiences." He thinks less than twice a month puts couples at risk for "more anxiety, tension and avoidance of their sex life."[37]

Once you come up with a mutually agreeable solution, schedule an opportunity for intimacy (I didn't say "have sex" here—there's no pressure, just prioritize the space to play) so the higher-desire person doesn't feel the need to badger and the lower-desire person can start anticipating it and not dreading it. Some days are off-limits, taking the pressure off until the planned schedule.

For the higher-desire partner, self-cultivation or nonpenetrative experiences with their partner (if they are willing, of course) can fill in for partnered PIV sex the rest of the time. That way, the higher-desire person isn't relying on the lower-desire person for all their orgasms, and the lower-desire person can start enjoying sex more knowing it is on a frequency that better fits their needs. Force-feed me ice cream and I will start hating ice cream. Let me choose what flavor and when. Now I am much more interested.

Important to note here: desire mismatch is a COUPLE problem, not an individual problem. In other words, he has a role in it, too. Engage and learn to communicate with him about it!

Pause and ponder these questions. Then discuss with your partner to see where your answers match and where they diverge.

- What comes to mind when you think about sex?
- What do you make sex mean (is it a "chore" or is it how you show/feel love)?
- Do you have/want "a lot" of sex? Why or why not?
- What is "a lot" of sex to you?
- What is a compromise that will make you both

happier? Why is this worth pursuing? You both don't have to be stoked. This is about what the relationship needs.

- What comes up when you ponder the idea of scheduling a block of time with each other where space may be held for intimacy, erotic touch, maybe massage or penetrative sex? How might that work for you? Does it take pressure off the other days?

- What do you want more of in your relationship that is not PIV sex? Cuddling, touching throughout the day, holding hands, a ten-minute check-in every night on the couch after the kids go to bed?

Other Factors

Oh, and here's another thought to consider: what you're feeling might not even be about desire at all. It might not even be about a problem YOU have! Often when women are asked why they have low desire, their answers point everywhere but to their own physical problems, like being in a strained relationship or their partner having erectile dysfunction.

But here's the thing: it's completely reasonable to not want to have sex with the partner you're having conflict with or divorcing! It's also completely common to be afraid to communicate about erectile problems and avoid sex as a result (even though it's not a great strategy, as we learned in Chapter Five: The Male Edition). None of that means you have low desire. It means you have no desire for a partner you've grown apart from, or no understanding how to expand your definition of sex to include more than just PIV activity. My bet is your sexual desire would return with an improved relationship or a guy who pays attention to your clitoris despite his ED.

In a study asking nineteen married women why they lost desire in their marriage, the three main themes discovered were:[38]

1. institutionalization of the relationship—a marriage that became rote or patterned. Remember what this does to dopamine, which loves novelty!
2. over-familiarity (becoming too familiar with a significant other literally is the opposite of eroticism and intrigue); and
3. the desexualization of roles in these relationships (mothering your spouse is NOT sexy).

Let's play this out a little further. Say you're an accomplished professional who works fifty-hour weeks, has two kids, and does the majority of the housework. You come home only to see x, y, and z still need to be done and the kids are going batshit crazy. If your husband asks for sex in that moment and you say no—does that make YOU the problem? Does that mean YOU have low desire? No. It most likely means you need help with the household and some time to transition off the cortisol that's making your stress levels soar before you can get in the mood. Sheesh. Barry and Emily McCarthy suggest that the most common cause of low desire is disappointment so if this scenario sounds familiar, please understand your lack of sexual desire is a natural consequence of the environment. It is not a "you" problem. (This is also a recipe for a very unhappy union.)

Now think about how different things would be if you came home to a clean house, a healthy meal waiting for you, and the kids already in bed. Your husband takes your coat and bag for you and says, "I took everything stressful off your plate. Let's make tonight about you. How can I help you feel relaxed?" That's sexy! That stokes desire! That just increased his odds of getting laid immeasurably!

As a physician, I hear so many women blaming themselves for low desire when that isn't what's actually happening. STAWP IT. You just need to find out what the problem REALLY is and address that. You got this!

CHAPTER ELEVEN

Desire Is SO Two-Faced

THAT "GOTTA-HAVE-YOU-RIGHT-NOW-OR-I-MIGHT-EXPLODE" excitement. Your body sending you thrills and chills telling you it's GO TIME. When just looking at your partner gets you thinking, *Yeah, let's do this!*

Wait, what? That doesn't sound like you? Or at least not the in-a-committed-relationship, older and wiser you? The adulting, working, parenting, not-quite-as-young-and-reckless-as-you-used-to-be you?

Relax! You didn't somehow "lose" your sexual desire like you lost that expensive pair of sunglasses last summer. What you're feeling—or rather, not feeling—is totally normal.

That's because there are actually TWO types of desire: spontaneous and responsive. Who knew, right? Well, I did only recently because I became a sexual medicine expert. But I didn't learn this in medical school, so doctors don't even know this.

Spontaneous desire is that Hollywood, pop/country hit, "desperately seeking" kind many of us experience at the beginning of a new relationship, especially as young adults when our testosterone and estrogen are at an all-time high. You start thinking about sex and go actively pursuing it.

Responsive desire, on the other hand, is when you're not having sexy thoughts crop up but once you get around to touching, kissing, and being naked and you're like, *I forgot how awesome this is!* as you are actively being sexual. Desire kicks in at different times in the process, but both end in the same result.

Spontaneous desire is considered the default in our society. Makes sense, because it's the MALE default and sex sells. The FEMALE default, though—especially in long-term relationships, when we have full, busy, multitasking lives, and as we age—is responsive desire.

Ever wonder why, as things evolved from hooking up/uncertain/ it's complicated to fully committed, your desire to have sex with your partner changed? That's because you transitioned from spontaneous to responsive desire. Spontaneous desire thrives on novelty, uncertainty, and new relationship energy (NRE). *Oooh, we've never done THAT before! I wonder if we'll see each other again? Does he want me? I wonder what x, y, and z with him will feel like.* Once the oxytocin and dopamine release associated with the novelty and uncertainty of new love goes away—which typically happens between six months to two years into a relationship—spontaneous desire hits the road and responsive desire takes over. Normal. Common. Just the way it is.

But I USED to have spontaneous desire, you might be thinking (insert judging yourself here). Unfortunately, having spontaneous desire for just one person forever isn't often a default thing. To get it back, you could leave your long-term relationship and find someone new...and then find someone newer when you lost it for them... and someone even newer after that...and so on and so on and so on. Basically, you'd need to replace your partner as often as twice a year to maintain spontaneous desire. But our society values long-term relationships, and I think a lot of us do too.

So maybe it's more the IDEA of spontaneous desire you want than the actual thing. This is such good news. I think people who habitually "fall out of love" after one to two years may be confusing love with the experience of spontaneous desire and NRE, and no one taught them what normal brains do with spontaneous desire over time.

But sex used to be so easy back then, you might protest. My guess and research on memory recall suggests that you're just remembering the absolute highlight reel, and forgetting the worry about pregnancy, disease, dating insecurity, and whatever else fill-in-the-blank we had back then, too. Sex wasn't easier, it was just different. Like relationships, desire grows and changes over time. That's okay.

Hollywood and the male viewpoint try to sell us spontaneous desire as the norm for everyone, all the time, but that's simply not the case for women. When we're in long-term relationships with busy lives, we are literally not into sex until we're in it. Once we're in it, we remember how great it is.

I hope knowing that women primarily experience responsive desire makes you feel more empowered. I hope it allows you to stay open to the idea of sex even if you weren't actively seeking it. I hope it helps you remember how much fun sex can be, and will be again once you take an active role in making it sex worth having and owning your agency in this arena.

Here are some ways to stoke responsive desire so it can feel like spontaneous desire.

Use your imagination. Actively picture your

Saturday night date before it happens. Think about that new outfit you're going to wear, the awesome meal you're going to eat, and the incredible sex you're going to have afterwards. Just anticipating it can start the juices flowing and encourage the release of dopamine. Whatever we focus on, we create more of. You can create desire with your mind. Desire is a thought, and we have complete control over the thoughts we choose.

Read or listen to erotica. While men are often more visual when it comes to sex—like, they see boobs and it's automatically go time—women are very context- or story-based. We need a sexy scenario to feel that same motivation. Reading or listening to a story about a couple being intimate in an Instagram-worthy cabin in the woods can give us the jump start we need. The Rosy Wellness app is a great place to find erotic stories geared toward women (bonus points—it was created by a gynecologist, Dr. Lindsay Harper). So put your body or mind in a sexy context to stimulate desire.

Initiate sex. Take control and have at it. Start by starting, knowing that desire will probably follow (and if not, you can still have fun together). Go after the sex you want to be having. Take an active role, and don't just lie around and accept what is given. Daydream, write, and design the menu. Partnered sex is a team sport. If you are on the sidelines, you aren't in the game.

If the majority of your experience is responsive desire, you're not wrong, faulty, or broken. It's not that you don't find your partner attractive anymore or fell out of love with them. You don't need a pill, cream, or tantric incantations to get your desire back. This is simply the way women's minds and bodies work, so big hugs. Zero need for a self-shame spiral.

One thing you *can* do to stoke more desire in general: work on desiring your partner in all aspects of life. Appreciate how good they look exercising, how manly they are negotiating something, how fatherly they are with the kids. Desire and foreplay start every day when you wake up. Try actively thinking, *Wow! I'm thankful to have this guy who is choosing to share this life with me. He works really hard to provide for our family.* He doesn't need to be perfect to be lovable or to have great sex with him. Gratitude and craving what you already have are superpowers.

When I was in residency, there was a general surgery resident who was married to an orthopedic surgeon. She would go around saying, "My husband is the hottest thing." She seemed to truly adore him. Seeing what those positive affirmations created in my friend's life, I actively chose to do what she was doing. Now anytime I talk about my husband, I always say, "He's so great. He's so hot." It won't work if you're lying, but giving attention to the good in our partner pays dividends in and out of the bedroom. My coaching teacher Brooke Castillo says, "Your thoughts about your marriage ARE your marriage."

A study in Australia in 2008 showed a woman's negative feelings about her partner was the most significant predictor of her level of sex-related distress, more so than age or menopause status.[39] So often women feel they need to change their partner, and most people don't want to change—us included, right? I think this comes from society never allowing us to be ourselves. We're always told we need to change, conform, or live up to an ideal, and this "never good enough" message trickles down and we end up saying the same thing to other people, especially our significant other and kiddos. My parents always wanted to change each other, and I think that was a big reason for their divorce.

Finding fault with your partner and then expecting your body to desire them is not how it works. You don't desire things you take for granted. Are you taking your partner for granted? Instead of trying to change him, support him in becoming the best person he can possibly be. In addition, mothering your partner is not good for desire.[40] Mothers aren't sexual with the objects of their mothering. Watch the roles you play with one another.

While the trade-off of being in a relationship is having spontaneous desire pack up and go, the good news is that sex can be hotter than ever with your long-term partner—especially when you're cultivating good thoughts about them. Expert after expert tells us that it takes years to get really good at sex. Michael Metz and Barry McCarthy, in their book *Enduring Desire,* point to research that shows the best sex occurs in couples who have been together for fifteen years or longer.[41] Other studies back this up, showing "women in relationships up to about ten years reported less sexual satisfaction and in later years (twenty-five to fifty) more sexual satisfaction than men at the same duration points."[42]

Grab a pen, take out a sheet of paper, and write down twenty-five things you desire. I'll wait.

Okay, how many things on your list do you already have—and if you're not desiring what you already have, why not? This is the body you have. This is the partner you have. This is the food in the kitchen you have. This is the life you have. Use it. Enjoy it. Live it. LOVE it. Desire it.

It is a myth to think you can only desire something you don't have. You can choose to desire what you do have. And when you do, it's MAGIC.

CHAPTER TWELVE

Brakes and Accelerators

DOES IT EVER feel like you can find a million reasons why you SHOULDN'T have sex, and very few why you SHOULD? If yes, it's no surprise. Society does its best to ingrain that kind of thinking into women, and we need to find ways to stoke sexual interest despite what we've been taught and told.

The Kinsey Institute was the first to develop the Dual Control Model of Sex. It theorizes that there are two independent systems controlling sexual arousal: The sexual excitation system (SES), and the sexual inhibition system (SIS). In her excellent and highly recommended book *Come as You Are*, Emily Nagoski refers to these as "the brakes and the accelerator."

Speeding Up

The SES, or accelerator, is what gets you in the mood for sex, or what tells your brain that something sexually relevant is around. Some accelerators might be a sexy story, a guy with a five o'clock shadow, watching your partner parent, laughter, a good meal, or being relaxed and stress-free in a hotel or a place other than the normal, boring, context of day-to-day life. These tell you *right now is an appropriate time to reproduce and feel good.* (BTW, very few people actually have sex to reproduce. Data from 2019 shows the average woman in America has 1.7 children, so there's not actually a lot of reproducing going on in a six-plus decade sex life.)

Typically, men are given free rein on the accelerator. They're conditioned to see your butt in those cute leggings and immediately want to hit the sheets, even though you just finished working out and need to shower, and the kids are still waiting to be fed. We can also rev things up by paying attention to our accelerators—the problem is most women were never taught to do that. Guess what? The path here might be simple: getting or giving a massage. Skin-to-skin contact. Touch that doesn't necessarily need to lead to sex, like holding hands, hugging, kissing in the morning, just sitting next to each other on the couch. Going on a date, laughing, dancing, reading erotica, or trying a new position. Emotional intimacy is a big accelerator.

Does a certain vibrator do it for you? Watching a sexy video? Having your partner take care of all the housework, put the kids to bed, and say, *Tonight's just about you, baby?* Doing thirty minutes of yoga and breathing to drop into your body and parasympathetic (calm, quiet mind) nervous system? Using a fantasy or connecting purposefully with your partner to relish being vulnerable or in charge in the bedroom? Your very fun assignment is to find out.

Adding accelerators when there's a trust issue in the relationship or one partner feels undervalued and taken for granted is a harder thing to accomplish. As the saying goes, foreplay starts at 8:00 a.m. How we treat each other the other twenty-three hours and thirty minutes a day is as important, if not more so, than our skills in the bedroom.

Slowing Down

The SIS, or brakes, is everything that makes you NOT want to have sex at the moment. The kids are still awake. There's no lock on the door. The neighbors might hear. You need to get to work. You're making dinner. Your sleep sucks, you don't love your body, you don't exercise, you think self-cultivation is bad, and society says sexually confident women are whores. Brakes tell you now is DEFINITELY not the time.

Brakes aren't bad per se, just like accelerators aren't always good. Even though it might seem like having our accelerators on all the time would be awesome, consider the downside. Having sex at work is not good. Sleeping with multiple people when you want to be in a monogamous relationship is a recipe for disaster. We can't just be having sex all the time or we'd probably starve and/or go broke (remember—our frontal lobe literally shuts off with orgasm). Our brakes prevent us from having too much accelerator.

Why do women get stuck braking all the time? The first unsurprising reason: society tells us we should brake. We're constantly fed BS like, *Don't have sex too much or you're a slut. Don't dress too sexy or you'll attract the wrong kind of attention. Sex is bad; it will get you pregnant and give you diseases. Women shouldn't desire, they should be desired. Sexual assertiveness isn't sexy.*

Second, we're made to feel like we have to do everything ourselves. For instance, we're not supposed to expect—no less ask for—help with childcare or around the house. That's just another brake, not an accelerator. In *Rising Strong*, Brené Brown says, "The danger of tying your self-worth to being a helper is feeling shame when you have to ask for help. Offering help is courageous and compassionate, but so is asking for help. "We need help taking off our "brakes."

Third, cortisol and our sympathetic nervous system (fight or flight) are brakes. When we are stressed and exhausted our bodies don't want to reproduce. We pack our lives full and run on caffeine, cortisol, and our sympathetic nervous system. What if all this sex life improvement stuff is just pointing us in another direction with how we run our lives? More parasympathetic, pleasure, and present moment are needed everywhere! And as Esther Perel says, "If you are too busy for sex, then you are too busy." Taking time for self-care isn't selfish. It is regulating.

Finally, there may even be an evolutionary component to it. It takes a lot of calories, vulnerability, and health risks to be pregnant, give birth, raise a kid (as those of us who are moms know all too well!). With all that hanging over our heads, OF COURSE we have trouble getting turned on if the conditions aren't right to feel safe and protected. Only when the parasympathetic nervous system (rest and digest) is activated can we take off brakes.

A brilliant paper by Dr. Sari van Anders et al. released in 2021 literally blew my socks off. In it, the authors argue that a heteronormative society causes women to live with the brakes on all the time and that "heteronormative gender inequities are contributing factors to a woman's low desire."[43] The four main contributing factors are:

- inequitable divisions of household labor
- blurring of partner and mother roles
- objectification of women
- gender norms surrounding sexual initiation (when the woman is only allowed to respond to the male's initiation, she doesn't have any opportunity to experience her own wants and desires.)

I was literally shouting out on the couch when I read this paper, "THIS! This is what women are living!" I've since had Dr. van Anders on my podcast. She is brilliant and I encourage you to listen to our chat!

Hitting the Gas

Having your brakes on in everyday life is perfectly normal. To prioritize your sexuality, you just need to stop stomping on them so hard and relearn how to hit the accelerator. Self- compassion goes a long way here as does curiosity towards yourself, your brakes, and your accelerators.

Everyone's brakes and accelerators are different. What might be a hard stop for one person might not even faze another. Some brakes are easy to address: bad breath is easily fixed; body odor gets washed away with a shower. But others aren't as quick to be reversed, like poor body image, thinking sex is "bad," having relationship troubles, or difficulty asking for childcare so you can have a weekend away to prioritize reconnecting.

It is common and normal for women not to be able to "light switch" from pre-frontal cortex, decision, house/job/kid management to sex (more on that in the next chapter). Take the time to ease off the brakes and turn on the accelerator. The more you work on what you need to transition, the easier and more natural it will get.

Not even sure what your accelerators are at this point? That's okay. While women are cultured and raised to have our brakes on, we're not taught to figure out what actually turns us on. That doesn't mean NOTHING puts you in a mood, it just means you haven't spent the time exploring what does.

After you've figured out what your brakes and accelerators are, communicate those with your partner. Teach them about the concepts of brakes and accelerators. Put a special focus on how you'd like to be approached to have sex. For instance, maybe it's a hard pass on your husband whining that you haven't done it in a week or grabbing your body as soon as you get home from work, and a super yes after he helps you out with everything that needs to get done in the house, makes you laugh, and speaks your love language.

Learn how to hit the gas together, and watch how your sex life went from coasting and avoiding to a lifelong adventure of self-discovery and communication. Now that you have learned about brakes and accelerators to your sexual life:

List your brakes.

List your accelerators.

Which was an easier list to make? Why do you think that is?

Next time you aren't "in the mood" understand why by listing the brakes that are on.

Can you intentionally find some accelerators to use?

CHAPTER THIRTEEN

Get Out of Your Head and Into Your Body

WE'RE CONSTANTLY MULTITASKING in the modern world. We do this, then that, sleep, get back up, and go do this and that some more. For better or worse, we take pride in this behavior. We make lists, try to check off as many things as we can as fast as we possibly can, and then start making more lists. Rinse, repeat, ad infinitum. Little do we know, the secret to getting turned ON lies in turning OFF this function.

But how many people do you know who feel like they always have to be *doing* something? Pretty much everyone, right? I'm going to let you in on a secret: it's okay to not "do" all the time. Sex, like life, is meant to be experienced, savored, and enjoyed. It's not just another cross-off-a-list kind of activity. If you think it is, well, you may have found a reason why it isn't enjoyable and meaningful.

Our list-making, task-loving, accomplishment-seeking selves live in the frontal lobe of the brain. But guess what *doesn't* live there? Sex. You can't be thinking about what you're cooking for dinner, how you need to get up tomorrow to x, y, and z, AND have an orgasm.

You have to tune out the everyday scanning and planning to tune in to pleasure. To get turned on, you have to turn off your mind and "drop into" your body. Dropping in means paying attention to the "down there" that includes everything that ISN'T the brain: your five senses, skin, breasts, butt, all the body, and the genitals. Experience your body in the moment, which is difficult if you let anxiety run the show or are observing and watching (a.k.a., judging) yourself have pleasure.

> "If you are depressed you are living in the past. If you are anxious you are living in the future. If you are at peace you are living in the present (and that is the only place orgasms live)."
> —LAO TZU (except the parentheses part by me)

The problem is that a lot of people look at sex as just another "frontal lobe" problem to solve: I just need to do it faster. I just need to change positions. I just need to buy a new toy. I just need to get it over with. Ugh, I just need to get some desire; why don't I enjoy it?

Everybody's looking for a quick fix, but it doesn't work that way. We look for a problem to "fix" when that in actuality IS the problem. It's so meta! All the sexperts will tell you that there is NO quick fix—not a supplement, lube, or vibrator (even though clitoral sonic air pulsation gadgets are pretty sweet). It is inner work, which is great news. There's nothing to buy and the solution is always free and available for life.

We act like our heads and our bodies aren't connected—like how people get pissed when a doctor tells them, "It's all in your head" (which really isn't meant to be offensive a lot of the time, though I digress)—but our brains and bodies are ONE. It is a Western paradigm to think they aren't connected. The truth is, they are always communicating.

So if you're stuck in your head thinking right now—and what you're thinking is, *I don't want to have sex; it's too hard, boring, gross, embarrassing*—it's time to acknowledge and work through your resistance. Is your mindset *I'm just having sex for my partner, I'm so not into it, I just want this to be over?* If so, you know what you're telling your body? That what's happening in the pelvis isn't pleasurable, and it isn't for you. You can't show up with resistance and expect it to be a wild ride of passion, relaxation, desire, and connection.

Even just noticing you're resistant to exploring your sexuality helps make space between your thoughts and reality. The truth is, you have agency over your own pleasure—and you're choosing to be resistant to it, rush it, or wish it was different. Maybe your thoughts are your "default" programming hardware and that feels totally permanent, like you can't change it. But you can, and that is where the work is for you.

To paraphrase Dr. Seuss, "Oh the places you can go!" Good news, you can change your default programming. Now where is that resistance coming from? Is it because your parents, religion, or culture told you sex was bad? That society told women to never be satisfied with their appearance? Just who are you bringing into the bedroom with you? No one needs their mom, an ex who told them their body wasn't perfect, the current spouse who tells them he will divorce them if their career gets bigger than his, or the judgy nun who taught high school whispering, *Bad girl!* in their brain when they're trying to enjoy themselves and connect with their partner. (I don't make these stories up, BTW—people can be shitty.)

Our bodies are perfectly capable of having pleasure. It is God-given—or evolutionary-given if that is more your thing—innate, within, a part of us, without us needing to choose it to be. We own a clitoris, for heaven's sake. It's our limiting beliefs that are limiting our sex lives. Sometimes the issue is in our heads. It's the psycho part of biopsychosocial.

Grab a sheet of paper and write down some not-so-positive beliefs about sex that you have in one column. In the second column, write where they came from (if you know). Notice how usually most of these thoughts aren't even yours. They were put there by somebody/something else. This can help us see that they aren't "real," and you don't own them any more than they own you. Part of the work is observing them and then letting them go.

Data shows women care about their male partner's orgasms more than their own.[44] How can you possibly relax into your body when you're thinking, *I'm taking too long,* like there's some universal sexual time limit? Or when you're "spectating" rather than being the person who's actually having the sex, wasting what otherwise could have been a good time thinking, *Is the light too bright? Is my butt too fat? Am I making a weird face? Is he having a good time?* Spectator thinking shuts down your ability to be successful sexually. Negative thoughts looping around your frontal lobe only take you out of your body more, and when that happens—orgasms are not on the agenda!

Mindfulness—some people like the term *awareness* or *presence* better—is necessary to take note of sexual triggers that occur in our day, and to pay attention to our accelerators and brakes. In *Running with the Mind of Meditation,* author Sakyong Mipham, a Tibetan lama and head of the Shambhala lineage, says, "The body benefits from movement, the mind from stillness." (I discovered this concept during my "how to change other people" phase of life. Ha, look what happened—I learned you can't change anyone but yourself.) Studies show sexual satisfaction increases by 60 percent when mindfulness is practiced. Put me in, coach!

Multitasking is a killer to sexual desire and arousal—and there's no better way to "get out of your body" than surfing on social media. I recently saw a statistic that said women check their phone up to ninety-six times a day and think about sex nine times a day. Clearly, we desire our phones more than sex by a long shot. What if we purposefully thought good things about sex more than we checked our phone? We have in our lives what we prioritize, right?

Seriously, don't be on the phone before sexy time. Sex can't compete with modern tech that was designed to steal our attention. In fact, research by SureCall, a manufacturer of cellular signal boosters, showed one in ten people checks their phones *during* sex!

The myth of multitasking is why busy, preoccupied women wonder why they don't have sex on the mind. Our mind literally can only do one thing at a time. If the brain is preoccupied with ANYTHING other than sex, it won't be interested in or as successful with sex.

As psychologist and female sexual arousal disorder expert Lori Brotto notes, "Research suggests that a woman's negative thoughts about her body pull her attention away from the erotic triggers and contribute to a lack of sexual arousal and desire." Working on self-image can make a big impact here. Studies show positive genital self-image results in less sexual distress and self-consciousness during sex, and is positively correlated with sexual desire.[45]

It's like "Goldilocks and the Three Bears":

- Paying no attention to your bodily sensations creates NO arousal
- Paying too much attention in a judgy and critical way kills arousal

- Paying just the right amount of attention but not in judgy way encourages arousal, curiosity, and enjoyment of the process

Just a little side rant here: SLOW DOWN AND ENJOY IT, PEOPLE! Why does everybody think they have to have an orgasm super freaking fast? Do you go to a nice resort and think, *Why can't I sit at this pool faster and be done with this experience? I wish my vacation would end quicker; I just want to get it over with.* Nobody says that! You're like, *I wish I could be here for a whole week* or *I want to live here!* What if we looked at sex like that? What if we considered it a special space to be enjoyed, not rushed? Then we would think, *This is lovely. I want this to last as long as possible!* Having a timeline for the speed of sex is "performative" sex, not pleasurable sex. Rushing or feeling anxiety about your timeline is simply not sexy, so slow down. If you literally have no time in your life for sex yet want or care about desire and a sexual relationship, I recommend really looking at your priorities. The average American spends two hours a day on social media and three hours watching TV—a lot of people have a lot of time! (And you working mothers: you might NOT have the time and I see you too! Don't add a "great sex life" to your to-do list right now. This may not be the season. Sex researcher Peggy Kleinplatz says, "People need to stop beating themselves up for not wanting to have sex when they have so much on their plates." You are busy. But when your schedule opens up, be mindful of saying NO to what you can and YES to whatever will enhance your pleasure and your relationship. The things we prioritize become our life.)

What you focus on during sex IS under your control, so here's a new thought to try: *My thoughts are optional, and they aren't facts. They can come and they can go.* You can observe your thoughts without hanging onto them. Yes, this is what the yogis and woo-woo influencers call mindfulness, but I promise you don't need a special cushion, repeat *ohm* for half an hour every day, or purchase your own secret mantra to get good at it. You can just realize, *Here I am thinking about my size again. That's curious, silly mind, but I'm not going to do that. Let's get back to oral sex.* Then take a big breath and drop back into your pelvis. This is what we call "nonattachment" to or "nonjudgment" of our thoughts: you have a thought, see it, and let it go. Yes, it takes training—but it will change your life, both in and out of the bedroom.

Remember, don't believe everything you think. Sex is a feeling thing, not a thinking thing. It is an experiencing thing, not a to-do thing. Tune out and become nonattached to that relentless chatter in your head. Tune back into your body's sensations, pains, needs, pleasure, and feedback.

As women, we're socialized to think our value is in what we do for other people. We're supposed to make sure everyone else is okay, but who's making sure we're okay? We can. We have to do that for ourselves.

Our needs do not come last. It's time we started prioritizing ourselves and our pleasure. Women do not exist on stress and coffee alone (nevertheless I tried for years; it is called surgery training, and turns out coffee is not a food group). All work and no play makes for a burned-out human.

You can start by trying to find joy in the everyday stuff. Practicing gratitude and looking for opportunities to accept play into your life. Providing your body with movement, going outdoors when possible, and listening to the sounds of nature. Savoring a hot shower or an awesome meal. There's a popular expression, sometimes attributed to Albert Einstein, which states, "There are two ways to live your life. One is as though nothing is a miracle. The other is as though everything is a miracle." If you can consistently take the stance that everything is a miracle, that mindset will follow you everywhere—including the bedroom.

Sure, I could give you a prescription for "how" to have great sex: number one, get undressed; number two, lie on a bed; number three, start touching each other...but does that sound fun? Think it will lead to a killer orgasm? Nope. It actually sounds awful. Like a chore. Just another thing to cross off your to-do list.

I want you to think of sex like a sport, body movement, musical instrument, or a craft instead. Get out there and practice. Get into it. See what works. The goal isn't perfection—if a golfer is thinking, *I need my next swing to be perfect*, it's definitely not going to happen and may actually get worse. The last thing anyone needs to be having is WORSE sex!

Professional athletes train their minds as much as their bodies. There is a lot of science behind getting out of your own way—and often, the obstacle IS THE WAY. Think of your main obstacle to enjoying your sexuality. Boom. That is where your work is.

The goal is simply pleasure and connection with another human when you are partnered, or with yourself when you are solo. That in and of itself is enough of a reason. We all deserve more pleasure in our lives.

Many people think that being a great lover is all about giving pleasure, but that is only half of it. Taking pleasure is just as important. Once you realize there's pleasure in the world and you are worthy of it, you can also receive pleasure. You can give pleasure to other people; people can give pleasure to you. You're as capable of giving and receiving pleasure as anybody else.

Bottom line: what you think about sex—or more accurately, stop thinking about it (that it's hard, annoying, not fun, and you just want to be done with it)—changes everything. There's no need to overanalyze things. As Timothy Leary once advised a bunch of tripping hippies: tune in (to your body), turn on (your clitoris), drop out (of your frontal lobe).

Okay, maybe he didn't say it that way, but it's probably what he meant.

CHAPTER FOURTEEN

Change Your Mind, Change Your Life

S EX IN AND of itself is neutral—it's our THOUGHTS about sex that can take us down a disaster of a rabbit hole. That's because thoughts (beliefs) lead to feelings, feelings drive actions, and actions lead to our results. Sex is a neutral circumstance (yes, one with a heavily loaded history of both abuse and splendor piled on top). It is only when the idea of sex is passed through our brain that we create context, meaning, and a "feeling" and "thought" about sex.

Here's an example: when you think, *Sex is hard and I'm not good at it and I don't desire/like it,* that leads to feelings of resistance, avoidance, and disdain. Those thoughts create the result that sex is a chore, so you don't go into the experience curious or relaxed or open. Your actions—the lack of enthusiasm and excitement about sex—are driven by those beliefs and lead to unsatisfying encounters.

Basically, it was predestined that you weren't going to have a good time because your thoughts already told your brain that was what would happen, and it played out from there.

This is why uncovering our thoughts about sex can go a long way toward changing our relationship to the circumstance of sex. New thoughts create different feelings that drive actions and produce the results we want. Thinking sex is boring, it takes too long, you don't desire it, and it's something you have to do leads to WAY different results than if you believe sex is fun, it's part of a healthy relationship, and you are a sexually confident woman who gets to have sex how and when she wants to.

The brain loves being right and always looks for evidence to confirm our limiting beliefs. Telling yourself you don't have time for sex makes your brain go, *That's so true—let me prove it to you! The kids require so much of your time. You have to do most of the housework. You have to go to work. You still have to find time to exercise.* But time scarcity is just another thought. You can actually find the time for sex if you think sex is important. Thinking, *Sex is important to me and my partner,* makes your brain say, *We're going to block some time on Sunday at 2:00 pm when the kids are napping because intimacy with you is a priority for me.*

Whatever you believe is going to happen is much more likely to happen, so it's important to clean up any thoughts that might block your enjoyment. You create your reality by how you think about sex. In other words, your sex life is a result of your beliefs, feelings, and actions.

For instance, a patient with a history of pain with sex due to endometriosis came to my clinic. Her condition was now under control and she wanted to get back into sex. My advice was to go into it with curiosity. I told her to cultivate thoughts like, *I wonder what's going to feel good*, instead of, *I know it's going to hurt*. Her brain was then primed to find pleasure instead of anticipating pain. Mindset matters!

Write down the top five things that you think are "blocks" for you from having the sex life of your dreams. Now, instead of thinking of them as barriers or excuses, they are your to-do list of homework to solve. Voilà! You just found your work and your five-step plan. The obstacles are the way.

Once you've worked on your thoughts, move on to your feelings. I want you to actually feel them using awareness and mindfulness. What a concept, right? All too often, we buffer our feelings with food, drinking, and overwork in an effort NOT to feel them. But even "bad" feelings (BTW, feelings aren't bad or good; we just label them that way) will pass if we don't resist them. Anger comes and goes; joy comes and goes; desire comes and goes. Feelings are just sensations felt in the body. No one died from feeling a feeling, but they do die from trying to AVOID feeling them.

Yes, desire can be both a thought and a feeling. If our thoughts are negative about desire—like, *I'm not worthy, I don't have desire,* or, *My partner is not worthy*—then the feeling of desire becomes much less available to us. Thinking, *I lost my desire,* is very disempowering. It takes you out of the driver's seat and puts you back on the sidelines. Everything we do or don't do in our life is because of how we think it will make us feel. We have evolved to do three things (this is known as the motivational triad):

1. move toward pleasure
2. avoid pain
3. conserve energy

And guess what? If we are doing numbers two and three, we aren't doing number one.

Interestingly, research shows that women with low desire have increased brain activity in parts that survey, judge, monitor ("spectatoring" as described by Masters and Johnson), and suppress emotions—so feel those feelings![46] Describe where the feeling is in your body. What are you feeling? What is happening in your body? What's going on now? Where is it now? Stay with it until it is processed and moves out of your body.

When we change our thoughts and feelings, our actions and results follow suit. Sounds easy, but it's not. The brain's number one priority is to keep us safe and survive, and change threatens this.

Growth only comes when you make a commitment to do the work. In this case, that includes changing your beliefs about sex, yourself, and your partner as well as your belief in your own capabilities. You have to be prepared to feel some discomfort and move toward it anyway.

Here's an example: we don't talk to our partners about sex because we want to avoid the discomfort that may come up. Avoiding talking creates its own discomfort in the form of a suboptimal sex life. The discomfort happens either way. Choose your path and know discomfort doesn't mean anything has gone wrong. The discomfort needs to be seen, felt, and processed. You can do this!

Share your wants and desires with your partner. A study by Uzma Rehmann et al. in 2011 demonstrated that sexual self-disclosure or communication about one's likes and dislikes in the bedroom is significantly associated with sexual satisfaction and function for both men and women.[47] Remember, if you always do what you've always done, you'll always get what you always got. Good sex takes time and practice. Curiosity and communication go a long way!

A common mistake here is action copying—doing things other people who have the results you want do—without changing the thoughts and beliefs behind the actions. But buying a vibrator, trying a new position, and scheduling sex won't change your sex life if you're still thinking sex is a chore and a bother. Making changes from the mind level leads to getting the results you want.

Here's where things get even more awesome. You can apply the concept of *change your mind, change your life* to ANYTHING—money, relationships, goals, your work environment. Uncover the thoughts that are holding you back to create the feelings and actions that will generate results like never before. To really get a hang of this, find a coach who can help you—resources are at the end of the book. Then, celebrate the badass you are!

Finally, stop should-ing all over your sex life. *I should have more sex. I should enjoy this type of sex. I should have an orgasm faster. I should lose twenty-five pounds first. I should have sex with him because he wants it even though I don't want it.* Let sex become the pleasure that it can be rather than something to beat yourself up over. Pressure and should-ing kill sexy every time.

We're lucky to have one thing in life meant just for the fun of it. Sex is adult play. ENJOY it. Try and learn. Get curious. It doesn't have to be so serious all of the time. Undo the passive thought of, *I'll wait around for desire to come to me.* Desire is not going to blow in on the next breeze. It is an active, participatory activity. Own your desire you create in the world. And what a radical idea to insist that your life be fun!

Don't accept the "low desire" label if that's not truly what's going on with you. Dig down deep to find the thoughts that are preventing you from having great sex. Work on your mind and watch how your body responds.

Your desire is literally within you. It never left you. Go inward to find it.

CHAPTER FIFTEEN

What a Pretty Pink Pill Can (and Can't) Do for You

O KAY, MAYBE YOU WEREN'T relieved when you read about the difference between spontaneous and responsive desire earlier in this section—because you can't find either of them these days and you aren't ready or willing to absorb the fact that desire isn't even necessary for a fantastic sex life. Maybe you've tried all the #lifecoach mind-body hacks I've suggested so far and still feel like things aren't working the way they're supposed to. (Remember that rewiring the brain and body takes a while.) Maybe you're even yelling at me right now, "Dr. C, I have ZERO desire. I truly think I have a medical PROBLEM!"

Fair enough. Let's take a deeper dive into hypoactive sexual desire disorder (HSDD) to see if it resonates with what you're experiencing. With over a thousand published manuscripts citing it, the Female Sexual Function Index (FSFI) Questionnaire is considered the gold standard measurement tool for doctors and therapists to diagnose HSDD. It consists of nineteen questions that address six domains of sexual function: desire, arousal, lubrication, orgasm, satisfaction, and pain. A score less than twenty-six indicates sexual dysfunction (even though they state that this is not a diagnosis calculator, only an indication that further questioning should happen).

I have a very happy sex life, and I scored 26.3—just barely above their cutoff for dysfunction. This was mostly because I didn't score high on the spontaneous desire questions (you get five points for "always or almost always" feeling sexual desire or interest). Um, excuse me? I work a high-stress, lots of hours, unpredictable job, and I still need to eat (and prepare said food), mother, and adult. Since we now know spontaneous desire is not the gold standard for females in long-term relationships (and that desire is not even a necessary component to have a satisfying sex life), I think this tool is biased toward the male default. Still, this is the tool that the experts agreed upon, so I will continue.

The other desire question is, "Over the past four weeks how would you rate your level of sexual desire or interest?" Again, if you have totally normal responsive desire, you would be docked points on this evaluation.

The International Society for the Study of Women's Sexual Health (ISSWSH) defines HSDD as "the persistent or recurrent deficiency or absence of sexual fantasies and desire for sexual activity with marked distress or interpersonal difficulty not otherwise accounted for by a general medical or psychiatric condition...lack of motivation for sexual activity as manifested by either reduced or absent spontaneous desire (sexual thoughts or fantasies) or reduced or absent responsive desire to erotic cues and stimulation or inability to maintain desire or interest through sexual activity or loss of desire to initiate or participate in sexual activity, including behavioral responses such as avoidance of situations that could lead to sexual activity...combined with clinically significant personal distress that includes frustration, grief, incompetence, loss, sadness, sorrow, or worry."[48]

What the FSFI doesn't measure is distress. So what if you score low on the lubrication questions? As long as you use lube and aren't distressed, it's not a barrier to having a good sex life.

Here's something else that's interesting to ponder: in a large population-based survey of more than fifty thousand women, almost 40 percent of participants reported having low desire—but only 10 percent said they were distressed about it.[49] The survey they filled out said low desire was a problem, but if they aren't bothered by it, maybe it's NOT a problem. Just saying. Again, there is no actual definition of "low desire."

Doctors also use the following screening tool for HSDD. To be diagnosed, you have to say yes to the first four questions and no to everything on question five.

1. In the past was your level of sexual desire or interest good and satisfying to you?	Yes/No
2. Has there been a decrease in your level of sexual desire or interest?	Yes/No
3. Are you bothered by your decreased level of sexual desire or interest?	Yes/No
4. Would you like your level of sexual desire or interest to increase?	Yes/No

5. Please check all the factors that you feel may be contributing to your current decrease in sexual desire or interest:

☐ An operation, depression, injuries, or other medical condition

☐ Medication, drugs, or alcohol you are currently taking

☐ Pregnancy, recent childbirth, menopausal symptoms

☐ Other sexual issues you may be having (pain, decreased arousal or orgasm)

☐ Your partner's sexual problems

☐ Dissatisfaction with your relationship or partner

☐ Stress or fatigue

It's pretty specific criteria. Most of us would check at least one factor listed in #5. For instance, many symptoms of menopause—decreased lubrication, hot flashes, and poor-quality sleep—contribute to low desire (and yes, there is help for all this that doesn't involve medication for low desire).

Overall Health Matters

Still think you have HSDD? Still want meds? Okay, let's forge ahead.

Doctors don't write prescriptions willy-nilly before they get to know a patient's history, so let's start with a few questions.

- How's your overall physical health?
- How's your social support network?
- Do you exercise?
- How's your mental health?

- Do you have any medical conditions?
- What medications are you taking?
- Do you smoke or drink alcohol?

Why does any of that matter? Because desire does not exist in a bubble. The healthier your body is, the more energy it has to expend on fun and pleasure. And sex = fun and pleasure.

Studies show following the Mediterranean diet, exercising, and maintaining a normal BMI all contribute to increased sexual desire and satisfaction. Are you doing some of that? Can you start? I cannot emphasize enough the role of taking good care of yourself when it comes to desire and sexual satisfaction. People with healthy bodies may find it easier to enjoy satisfying sex lives as sex is a physical activity. (For example, the Olympic Village is apparently a total sexfest, with endorphins and peak physical forms everywhere. At the 2021 Tokyo Olympics, one hundred sixty thousand condoms were handed out to eleven thousand Olympic athletes—and no one else is allowed in the village. You do the math.) Yes, all bodies can enjoy good sex and should, but there is something to not feeling tired all the time and instead feeling strong and with good endorphins flowing through you that really helps sex.

SUPERCHARGE YOUR SEX LIFE WITH EXERCISE

Research shows women who exercise and have a healthy body image have more sex and more enjoyable sex. Need more reasons to get up and get moving? Exercise has been shown to:

- Improve body image and self-esteem. Data shows people who exercise feel better about themselves and feel they are more sexually attractive than people who don't exercise. Our thoughts about our bodies and our desirability are huge—so rock on with your sexy exercising self!

- Prevent erectile dysfunction and sexual dysfunction in women—especially cardiovascular exercise. A 2021 study looked at women who had come to a clinic for sexual dysfunction. They found participants who did four to six hours of physical activity a week showed better sexual function and clitoral vascularization, lower sexual distress, and reduced odds of having HSDD and genital arousal disorder. Interestingly, the women who did more than six hours a week of exercise had worse sexual function. The authors believe this was more related to body image issues—which, remember, is a killer to sexual health and function—than the exercise itself.[50]
- Can help stimulate arousal—research has shown improvements after a single bout of exercise. The more fit you are, the better blood flow you have—and we need blood flow to engorge our erectile tissue and push fluid through the vaginal wall for lubrication (man, have I won an award yet for making sex not sound very sexy?).
- Decrease joint pain discomfort, which is a sexually limiting problem as we age.
- Increase muscle strength and endurance—and the stronger your pelvic floor is, the more intense orgasms are supposed to be.
- Reduce stress—stress is a total turnoff. Stress makes you exist in that sympathetic "fight or flight" nervous system. This is so bad for enjoying sex.

Social support is also a huge contributor to desire (or lack thereof). When you have other creative outlets that fill your needs beyond your primary relationship, your mind and body realize, *It's safe to get sexy! I've got what I need!* Data shows that having a great network of friends and family is correlated with a happy sex life. Do you have the support and connection you need?

The same is true for having a supportive partner that shares in an equal amount of housework. There is even a study showing men who do an equal amount of household chores have more sex because they are helping "take the brake off" the cognitive and physical load of our to-do list that prevents interest in sex. "When male partners reported making a fair contribution to housework, the couple experienced more frequent sexual encounters, and each partner reported higher sexual satisfaction one year later."[51]

On the opposite end of the spectrum, medical issues detract from desire. As I've mentioned before, smoking causes erectile dysfunction in men and low arousal due to decreased blood flow in women. Unfortunately, pelvic radiation and surgery do the same. There is also plenty of data that poor sleep, stress, physical inactivity, being overweight (clinically, like in a metabolic-syndrome and glucose-intolerant way, not in the luscious, sexy-at-any-size way), and having diabetes, heart disease, anxiety, and/or depression sinks your sex life.

I recently had a patient come to see me for low desire. She also had diabetes, anxiety, and depression, didn't exercise, and her weight was not heart-healthy. When I asked what she wanted—what she wished would happen—her answer was, "I don't know." I think she secretly hoped I could give her desire, but desire isn't going to magically appear when someone isn't taking care of their body and mind (not two separate things, remember). Think of sex as expendable. When the body has other priorities like mental health, inflammation, and exhaustion to deal with, sex is an expendable event. It is not necessary for continuing your life (just the life of the species). Another question she couldn't answer was, "What kind of sex do you want to be having?" so I recommended she start by asking herself, "What kind of sex do I NOT want to be having?" Reverse engineer your sex life this way.

Journal time: what kind of sex do I NOT want to be having?

Mental health issues—25 percent of Americans deal with this—can really do a number on desire, too. If you carry around chronic anxiety, of course that's going to impact whether you want to have sex or not. Anxiety is a huge brake (and definitely not an accelerator) for your sex life.

The highest prevalence of HSDD is seen in women between the ages of forty and sixty-four who are: partnered, sexually inactive, more educated, and/or taking psychotropic medications. Urinary incontinence and pelvic organ prolapse are also associated with female sexual dysfunction. A study showed women with urinary incontinence and/or urinary tract symptoms complained of sexual dysfunction, with 34 percent reporting HSDD, 23 percent sexual arousal disorder, 11 percent orgasmic deficiency, and 44 percent sexual pain.[52] Midurethral slings (or transvaginal tapes, as they are sometimes called) to prevent bladder leakage consistently show improved sexual function, likely through the boost of confidence and improved self-image they provide women by helping to not leak urine. This benefit continued even years after the surgery.

However, no surgery in the pelvis is without risks. Sling surgery requires going around the inside part of the clitoris and making a midurethral incision that's close to the sexually pleasurable urethral-clitoral erectile tissue. As such, very rarely it could cause further sexual dysfunction. In my practice, I don't often see sexual issues after slings, but all of my sling consent forms list sexual dysfunction as a rare but real risk. I believe women need to know pros/cons of any surgery they agree to. If you are a candidate for this procedure, talk to your doctor about the advantages and risks associated with it.

Urethral bulking is the new kid on the block to help stress incontinence. And don't forget about pelvic floor physical therapy. Both are effective for bladder leakage and don't require mesh tape insertion. Talk to your local friendly urologist or uro-gyn surgeon to determine the best options for your situation.

So why did I spend this much of a "medication chapter" talking about health first? Because the last thing I want is for you to try and fail medication and then end up feeling even more broken. Promise me you're going to work on any underlying causes that may be contributing to your low desire—even if you choose to pursue a prescription medication to help boost it. Just because you're taking a high blood pressure pill doesn't mean you shouldn't also exercise and work on your diet and stress, right? The same holds true here.

Medications for Low Libido

Okay, NOW it's time to hear all about the medications that are FDA approved in premenopausal women to treat HSDD, as well as some other off-label ones. Finally, right? And sorry, there are NO medications that are FDA approved to treat postmenopausal women for low desire, at least not yet. Ageism? Likely.

The two FDA-approved drugs for HSDD in premenopausal women are:

1. VYLEESI (BREMELANOTIDE)

This acts on the melanocortin receptor to increase spontaneous desire (melanin, which creates pigmentation of the skin, is also regulated by these receptors). To use Vyleesi, you inject it forty-five minutes before anticipated sexual activity. It has been shown to increase desire and decrease distress slightly but does not change the number of sexually satisfying events per month. When using Vyleesi, 40 percent of users experience nausea, 4.8 percent vomiting, and 3 percent cough. (I tried it and coughed for four straight hours. Not sexy, and also not possible to have sex when you're coughing like that. Like any good researcher, I tried it again. Repeat coughing. Epic sexy fail for this scientist. Amused hubby in the wings—what a good sport.)

While studying bremelanotide's effectiveness as a sunless tanning product, one of the researchers decided to take a double dose. It gave him an erection for twenty-four hours! So they decided to see if it had any sexual benefits for women. Yup, it did.

2. ADDYI (FLIBANSERIN), A.K.A. THE "LITTLE PINK PILL"

By decreasing serotonin and increasing dopamine and norepinephrine in the brain, Addyi brings glutamate levels down to help users drop out of their frontal lobe and into their body. (In HSDD, high levels of glutamate overstimulate the "multitasking area" of the brain and make it hard to shut off.) It has been shown to increase the number of satisfying sexual events (SSEs) per month by about one half over placebo in all women, but in the "true responders" it increased SSEs by five per month. (Remember, sexual events is not our goal; enjoying desire and sex is—the researchers chose to measure "events" as they are easy to count and therefore quantify.) In terms of side effects, 11.4 percent of users experience dizziness, 11.2 percent somnolence, 10.4 percent nausea, and 9.2 percent fatigue (which I guess is not too bad if you have trouble sleeping!). Flibanserin is a daily drug and may take a few months to notice a difference. Dr. Rachel Rubin, a fellow rock-star urologist and sex ed expert, says, "When we add dopamine in the brain, people have more desire. These medications don't work for everyone, but like any medicine that works on the brain, it can work in about 50 to 60 percent of people and it can work really well. I have so many patients who just have sexual thoughts, which gives them so much satisfaction and hope. Plus, we have seen no risky side effects from this medication. What is the harm in trying it if the patient is looking for a biopsychosocial approach?" We use meds to treat depression. And therapy. Both together are a great combo. We can think that way about these meds, too. Dr. Rubin reminds us, "How can you change your mindset when you are disgusted by the idea of sex? If a pill lifts that fog, you will be more open to working on your mindset."

Addyi was originally being tested as an antidepressant drug. Women weren't less depressed when they took it—but they DID want to have sex more. So it became an HSDD drug instead, and here we are.

A note here: while premenopausal women have two FDA-approved meds for sexual health and postmenopausal women have zero, men have many more—not even including testosterone. It turns out, the panel tasked with approving flibanserin was made up of solely male physicians, none of whom had ever treated women for sexual dysfunction. They somehow decided pre- and postmenopausal women were different enough and only approved it for the former group. It should be noted that there were no studies showing these medications are unsafe for postmenopausal women.

Not to worry. You can still get a prescription even if you're in menopause—it will just be considered off-label. "Off-label" is just another way to say "your insurance may not cover it." The reality is, it may not be covered even if you are premenopausal, as many insurances exclude sexual health medications (which is fine if you own a penis and generic Viagra is two dollars a pill or less, but not so much if you're a woman who has to pay hundreds for Addyi or Vyleesi). Consult your doctor about a specialty pharmacy (or the drug's website or the drug representative) to find the cheapest option. You can often get a discount or free month's supply while you see if the medication works for you.

So is an FDA approved med for low desire too good to be true? Perhaps. Reason number one: these meds aren't curative, meaning you have to keep taking them to keep having an effect. Reason two: a meta-analysis of eight trials and 5,941 women on flibanserin showed that satisfying sexual events increased, on average, by 0.49 per month compared with placebo "while statistically and clinically significantly increasing the risk of dizziness, somnolence, nausea, and fatigue." Scores on the six-point Female Sexual Function Index improved by just 0.27 points.[53] However, they DO help some people very well. We just haven't yet figured out who will benefit the most. Don't hear me as a total hater. I am not opposed to medication, I am just afraid a woman won't try to address her biopsychosocial component of her sex life, take a medication not understanding the role of desire, continue having shitty sex, and then pile on "medication failure" because the meds didn't work for her. That's all. So go for it if you want to. I have your back. If they don't work for you after three to four months of use you can stop.

What about those off-label medications I mentioned before? Here are a few others that might help HSDD that have not yet been approved by the FDA.

- **Oxytocin.** Studies on a small number of women have shown scores on the FSFI improved after using it in a vaginal gel form. Other studies show it doesn't work.
- **Cannabis.** Some studies suggest improved sexual function when using cannabis, specifically ease of orgasm.[54] Unfortunately, most of these are based on survey data, which is fraught with bias. Several studies also suggest an inhibition of sexual function. Likely, effects are dose dependent, and too much is probably not helpful.
- **Viagra (sildenafil).** This has been shown to help in women who have arousal issues but has not been proven to increase desire. It works by increasing blood flow to the genital tissues and penis = clitoris, so of course it would work in clitoris owners. Just remember desire does not equal arousal (nonconcordance) in most women. Researchers are working on a topical cream to help with women who need more blood flow secondary to medical conditions or aging. Stay tuned or try a compounded product.
- **Wellbutrin (bupropion).** This antidepressant is a bit different from other SSRIs that are most commonly used for depression. Studies show it improves sexual function but has no effect on frequency of sex. Research proves using it in conjunction with a current SSRI is effective in treating SSRI-induced female sexual dysfunction as well as increasing desire.
- **Buspirone.** This antianxiety drug works by decreasing serotonin. When added to a current SSRI, 58 percent of people saw an improvement in sexual function compared to 30 percent with placebo.[55]
- **Testosterone.** This works great for desire in perimenopausal and postmenopausal women. For women with low libido taking SSRIs, testosterone therapy resulted in a significant increase in the number of satisfying sexual events compared with placebo in women enrolled in a double-blind study.[56]

You may be asking yourself, *What about alcohol?*
That sometimes seems to help me get in the mood! I
am certainly not promoting alcohol use (it is a known
carcinogen linked to eight types of cancer including
breast and colon), but I also think you need to know the
good and the bad here.

On the positive side: when you drink alcohol,
it makes the brain not care about the past or the
future—exactly what mindfulness does. Not thinking
about anything but the present makes for better sex.
It can also help turn off brakes, letting all the reasons
you can usually think of to NOT have sex melt away. In
addition, alcohol is antianxiety and helps to diminish
sexual worries and inhibitions.

The negatives: alcohol creates brain myopia—
meaning a lack of foresight or intellectual insight—
which is one reason drunk people are much more
likely to engage in risky sexual behavior (their brains
are not thinking about tomorrow or how this could
be a bad idea in the future). It is depressant, which
can decrease sexual arousal by interfering with the
connection between the brain and genitals, and can
make orgasm take longer. It also causes poor sleep
and lowers libido by decreasing testosterone and can
cause vaginal dryness.

I'd say the bad outweighs the good here, but you're
an adult and can make your own decisions! #agency

So there you have it—the lowdown on what medications can and
can't do for your desire and arousal. See your doctor for a prescription if you meet the criteria for HSDD. Keep in mind that
while physicians are well-versed in Viagra—it has been around for

decades—they may not be trained in female sexual health. It's also important to realize the available FDA-approved medications do not work for everyone and have to be taken consistently to work, and all drugs can have icky side effects.

F*ck Desire?

I totally understand why you'd want to try that little pink pill dubbed as the "female Viagra" to get your sex life back on track—you want to make sex feel great and exciting again. Medicine seems like the easiest and best way to reignite your fire, right? Of course, now we know it's not that simple all the time. While pills can stimulate blood flow and release certain neurotransmitters in the brain, they aren't magic.

Americans take more pills than any country in the world (many of which are life-saving or at least life-improving, and I don't hate on all of them by any stretch). However, it is a result of our culture's belief that solutions lie in pills, and that we don't need to do the work of caring for our bodies, brains, and relationships. Any sexpert will tell you that sex is wonderful in its complexity and you miss the opportunity to grow, learn, and improve when you look for a quick external fix. Many don't like that the pharmaceutical industry is trying to monetize what society has sold women—that spontaneous desire is necessary and your body should work like a man's (because that is better).

I also wish HSDD wasn't seen as a binary, meaning you either have it or you don't. In my urology practice, I often see patients with sensitive bladders that are irritated by certain foods. When they come in and ask, "Do I have interstitial cystitis?" my answer is always, "Would you like a chronic, incurable disease to carry around with you forever?" When they inevitably say no, I tell them, "In that case, let's just say you have a sensitive bladder that doesn't like spicy food."

Desire comes and goes, and you might find yours yet. If you want to. Or, f*ck desire. Even if a pill could give desire to you, it isn't always necessary and doesn't guarantee a happy sex life either. You can have incredible sex without waiting for desire to come first. This is such a mind-blowing concept—but it is also incredibly freeing. Why make it harder or more complex than it has to be?

We often think: if I only had desire, I would have great sex and more romance. Nope, this is backwards! Research done in 2021 mining previous studies using machine learning found that higher sexual satisfaction and feelings of romantic love toward one's partner is the biggest predictor of sexual desire.[57] Literally no studies say desire is a predictor of sexual satisfaction. Sex and romance are what SPARK desire.

With things like food, water, and sleep, the less you have the more you want them. Sex doesn't work that way—there isn't that same kind of inherent drive toward it. For many women, the more we go without sex, the LESS we think we need or want it. In this way, sex doesn't act like our other nature-driven desires at all. Data shows that less sex leads to less sexual satisfaction, which leads to rejecting more initiations of sex by our partners.[58] (Which leads to even less sex. Which leads to ever greater unhappiness. It's a vicious cycle.)

Great sex truly isn't about libido and desire. The only problem is THINKING that's a critical component to get started. You can just decide that you want to have magnificent sex right now, problem solved. It will still take curiosity, communication, and practice, but desire isn't a necessary ingredient to start down this path.

Positive anticipation is the secret ingredient. Take care of that and here comes your desire. Shitty, unsatisfying sex does not cause positive future anticipation. Work on your sex life, and the desire will follow. I don't wait for desire to eat vegetables or exercise. I do these things because I want them in my life and I enjoy them during and after doing them. Find your WHY for your sexuality. Your WHY will change your motivation and therefore your sex life.

Embrace the Opportunity

Besides, what if your "low libido" is an opportunity? A doorway? A calling to find out where your ACTUAL desire lies? What makes you tick? What turns you on? What your relationship needs? What your stressful, fully packed lifestyle is asking from you? What if your low desire is a healthy response to unwanted, unenthusiastically consented, or lusterless sex?

> The term libido comes from Latin for desire or lust. Freud, in his early work dating back to 1894, used it to mean a psychic energy or primitive biological urge. Now we simply define it as sexual drive. Again, it is a very male-centric view of how sexuality works.

Maybe this is a wake-up call—your inner self whispering that you need to pay attention and change something in your life. Sometimes it will be the relationship you are in. Often women only see in hindsight, when their desire for sex and life comes raging back after the end of a twenty-year marriage that was stifling them.

Or perhaps this is so distressing because you feel you aren't being true to yourself. In *Hamlet*, Shakespeare wrote, "To thine own self be true." What do you need to learn from your "low desire" to be true to yourself? That you are stretched too thin, burning the candle at both ends, refusing to ask for help, saying yes to sex when you mean no, and doing everything yourself in an effort to be the perfect woman?

Don't box yourself in when you don't have to. There's no need to stick yourself with a label for life, like, *Oh, I'm the low-desire person.* This might just be a blip in time and not a permanent problem. Taking an active role in improving your sexuality is where the true personal and societal revolution lies!

It's time to knock down sex exceptionalism. Sex, just like every-thing else in life, doesn't have to be this big, challenging thing. Let's enjoy it and incorporate it into our lives without all the giant expecta-tions. Either work to cultivate more desire in your life, say f*ck desire and go have some great sex anyhow, or do both. It all ends up in fun.

Whatever you do, stop thinking you don't have enough desire. It's not a prerequisite for sex. You're perfectly normal!

In *Magnificent Sex: Lessons from Extraordinary Lovers*, Peggy Kleinplatz, PhD, states, "The overwhelming majority of extraordinary lovers told us that intercourse was irrelevant, inconsequential and/or unnecessary for optimal sexual experience." (But you already figured that out by now, right?) Her research determined that people who have magnificent sex:

- are master communicators and set aside time for the opportunity for erotic encounters
- let go of past beliefs that limit their pleasure, including body image and feelings of unworthiness to enjoying pleasure
- always have consensual sex
- say sex improves as their relationships improve and are fans of "trial and error" in figuring it out
- realize it takes dedication and practice to become fluent in their sexuality
- are able to "center themselves" to totally "inhabit the present moment"
- have significant empathy toward themselves and their partner
- foster trust, respect, and safety

CHAPTER SIXTEEN

Maybe It's Menopause

IF YOU'RE TEMPTED to skip over this chapter, don't. Why? Because if you are a woman who plans to live after fifty, or a man who cares about a woman who plans to live after fifty, you need to know what else is coming. The average age of menopause in America is fifty-one. With our current life expectancy, that means women now spend one third to one half of our lives in menopause. For that reason alone, it only makes sense to learn as much as possible about it—even before it happens—so we can make the most of those years and won't ever have to ask, "Why didn't anyone tell me?"

Menopause Basics

Let's start with the basics. You can start having symptoms of menopause—called perimenopause—in your late thirties and, rarely, sooner. Other women have their periods regularly into their late fifties without symptoms. There's just a huge range of experiences.

The technical definition of menopause is not having a period for twelve months. That can be confusing and less than inclusive, because a lot of women have IUDs, don't have periods for other reasons, or have had their uterus ablated or removed. We'll have to settle for it anyhow. No periods (with the exception of the above) is basically an outward sign that your estrogen is very low. How low? Lower than a man's, actually. So low that your body can't cycle or reproduce.

In twelve months and one day without having a period, congrats! You've reached menopause. Now what?

Again, women have a wide range of experiences. Some have all the classic symptoms: hot flashes, mood swings, disturbed sleep. These can last a few months, years, or even a lifetime. Other women have virtually none. Studies show hot flashes last about seven years, but many women continue to have them beyond that timeframe. This is a major quality-of-life issue. Hot flashes have been linked to increased risk of heart disease and poor sleep, which both lead to shorter lives.

Menopause and Sex

Here are two facts about menopause that are very important to us:

1. It is a myth that menopausal women have less quality sex. Studies show sexual satisfaction actually INCREASES with age. In fact, more than half of sexually active women over the age of eighty report sexual satisfaction happening "almost always." What is even more noteworthy in this study is that only 3 percent of the women surveyed said they felt sexual desire always or almost always.[59] Sexually satisfied women don't rely on desire!

2. The main reason postmenopausal women STOP having sex is a) vasomotor symptoms like hot flashes, night sweats, poor sleep, and vaginal dryness, and b) availability of their partner. As a doctor, I can't often help you with b.

Okay, so now I'm telling you that sex can be great in menopause and doesn't require desire as an ingredient, BUT it can also come to a screeching halt because of menopause symptoms. Never fear. Treatments for menopause symptoms have been around for decades. But the shroud of silence, fear, and shame keeps most women in the dark about how safe, cheap, and useful these treatments are.

FYI, testosterone replacement for postmenopausal women can have great benefits on our sex lives. Plenty of data shows it helps with desire and arousal. Unfortunately, testosterone replacement is not yet FDA-approved in this country like it is in Australia. Ask your doctor anyway—nearly 21 percent of prescriptions for branded male testosterone products are written for females. There are international guidelines to help guide your provider.[60]

Testosterone is only indicated for postmenopausal women. The theory is that premenopausal women still make enough of it naturally, so low testosterone is unlikely to be the cause of low libido. Another reason not to give to women who can still get pregnant is that testosterone is dangerous to a fetus. But if you are in your late thirties or older, it may be worth getting checked as perimenopause can start lowering testosterone. As with all medicine, there are likely some premenopausal women who may benefit. See a specialist for a comprehensive discussion as it relates to you.

Hormone Therapy Myths and Truth Bombs

Relief can come with hormone therapy (HT)—formerly known as hormone replacement therapy (HRT). Dr. Jenn Gunter explains why this new nomenclature is necessary in her book *The Menopause Manifesto*. Because the term has the word "replacement" in it, this "falsely implies that estrogen or other hormones are missing because of a medical problem, and the low levels of estrogen after menopause are biologically abnormal." Menopause is not a disease!

Are you thinking, *OMG, does she WANT me to get cancer and a heart attack and die just so I can keep having sex?* Of course not! What I want is for you to know that you've been sold a pack of lies about hormones that are just as big as the ones society taught you about sex.

Here is a "history of medicine" lesson to share with anyone who will listen. In the nineties, the Women's Health Initiative decided to study the protective effects of estrogen on heart disease to see if they could show that fewer women would die of heart disease (still our number one killer of women and men in America) if we put them on hormones. As part of their research, women in their seventies—who hadn't had estrogen since going through menopause twenty or more years earlier—were started on it. The study was stopped early after a small increased risk of breast cancer, cardiovascular disease, blood clots, and stroke was found among the women taking the hormones compared to placebo.

Of course, the media went wild. The headlines were sensational, claiming ESTROGEN IS BAD! Women were literally ripped off their hormones—70 percent of estrogen prescriptions in our country were stopped at that point—even though doctors had known for quite a while it was the best treatment for hot flashes, disturbed sleep, and mood changes due to menopause.

What's important to note here is that this study was NOT looking at the beneficial roles of estrogen during menopause transition (healthy women ages forty-five to sixty, or within ten years of the start of menopause). What we ACTUALLY learned from the Women's Health Initiative was older women shouldn't be thrown back on estrogen if they haven't had it for decades. And most doctors weren't even doing that in the first place in real-life medical practice!

The truth is, estrogen is heart protective. One theory why women get heart disease so much later than men is because it helps prevent plaque buildup in our arteries. Once estrogen goes away, though, our arteries do exactly what men's arteries do—they start collecting plaque. And if you throw estrogen back into the body in your seventies, those plaques get destabilized and may cause strokes, which is exactly what happened with the Women's Health Initiative. Today, there is even data that shows taking HT in "early menopause" is heart protective, while not using HT in younger menopause (before age forty) increases the risk of cardiac disease.[61]

With regard to estrogen increasing the incidence of breast cancer, that's just another misconception generated by the Women's Health Initiative. In their research, estrogen was actually shown to have a PROTECTIVE effect on breast cancer, but not enough to be recommended for prevention. It was participants who took a combination of both estrogen and progesterone that showed a very slight increased risk of breast cancer compared to placebo. Further analysis suggests this placebo group already had a very low risk of cancer—lower than the placebo arm in the estrogen-only group—because participants weren't randomized for their risk of cancer going into the study, which is very important in studies looking at causes of cancer, and some in the placebo group had previously been on estrogen (which decreased their risk of breast cancer, making the "treatment arm" look like a higher risk). And the ones who got cancer still lived longer than people with breast cancer who weren't on any hormones at all! Current experts agree that any risks of breast cancer with HT are negligible. Unfortunately, breast cancer is quite common and women will get it while on HT, but HT is unlikely to be the cause of it. Having a first-degree relative with breast cancer is not a contraindication to taking HT.

> If you really want to reduce your risk of cancer, don't drink alcohol (classified as a carcinogen by the World Health Organization in 1988—this is not new news even though less than half of Americans know that alcohol is cancer-causing) and keep your body mass index below thirty (BMI is an imperfect measure, I know, but visceral fat is inflammatory). Both of these carry a much higher risk of cancer of many types, not just the breast.

There is evidence for estrogen's role in sexuality as well. Estrogen replacement should be considered in all menopausal women (who are candidates for it) who present with sexual concerns, especially if they are symptomatic from menopause.[62] One study that looked at both hormones and relationship factors noted that estradiol is important in sexual responsiveness and desire, but also found that, "Prior function and relationship factors are more important than hormonal determinants of sexual function of women in midlife."[63] In other words, all the other stuff in this book is still really important—otherwise I would just slap an estrogen patch on everyone and call it a day. Don't forget our favorite way to view our sexuality: biopsychosocial!

The Women's Health Initiative Study was stopped and published in 2002, so it's taken twenty years for this conversation to get back to the facts: hormones are life-improving and very safe for many women. Estrogen (especially when given in young menopause, which is roughly considered before age sixty) protects against heart disease, anxiety and depression, breast cancer, colon cancer, cognitive problems, insulin resistance, and osteoporosis. Several studies have shown that hormone replacement increases longevity.[64] There is even data that says women who take HT live on average three years longer than women who don't.[65]

So why are women still suffering when we don't have to? One reason is that doctors stopped learning how to prescribe these FDA-approved medications, pushing women into the cash-based hormone clinics that use compounded hormones, check labs all the time, and cost an arm and a leg. I don't blame the women who go to these—they just want to feel better—but just know that data shows compounded HT (often given in pellets or injections) has higher side effects and risks than the FDA-approved products.[66] For that reason, the North American Menopause Society and the American College of Obstetrics and Gynecology do not recommend pellets or compounded hormones in most cases when safer FDA-approved products are available.[67] Buyer beware! Also, insurance pays for blood work that is medically necessary and FDA-approved medications. Treating your symptoms and getting the health benefits of hormones shouldn't break the bank.

The vagina and vulva are estrogen dependent. When our body isn't getting estrogen, a lot of uncomfortable things can happen. This is referred to as genitourinary syndrome of menopause (GSM), which includes:

- Vaginal dryness, itchiness, irritation, bleeding, and pain with sex. (True story: A patient of mine went to her regular doctor complaining of vaginal dryness and she was offered an antidepressant. When she asked, "Will that help?" the doctor said, "Probably not, but it might bother you less." People! This was in 2021! Antidepressants are NOT standard of care for vaginal dryness or menopause symptoms, but are commonly used. Feel free to get second opinions.)
- Decreased arousal (pelvic blood flow arousal, not to be confused with brain arousal)
- Difficulty reaching orgasm and clitoral shrinkage and phimosis (adherence of the hood skin to the glans)

- Burning with urination
- Increased urinary urgency and frequency, which is often treated as overactive bladder instead of GSM
- Recurrent urinary tract infections (UTIs). Vaginal estrogen decreases recurrent UTIs by up to 68 percent and is a recommendation in the American Urological Association's guidelines for UTI.[68]

Without hormones, vulvovaginal atrophy occurs in 50 to 80 percent of menopausal women, and it only gets worse the longer you go without them. The clitoris has less blood flow, collagen decreases, and the labia minora begins to resorb (in layman's terms, dissolve or go away)—a problem not only because it is a sexual organ that contains erectile tissue, but also because it protects the urethra from trauma. Once the "curtains" are gone, so to speak, UTIs and vaginal infections become a recurrent and painful issue for many. (I only found all this out at an ISSWSH meeting—before that, I thought maybe the older women I was examining had been born without labias!) I literally didn't learn this in medical school or during residency where I trained to be a pelvic surgeon.

Ready for some good news? All these symptoms can be alleviated by using either systemic or vaginal estrogen. Systemic estrogen is absorbed through your body by taking a pill or using a patch or ring. Vaginal estrogen is absorbed through the vagina and comes in the form of a cream, pill, or ring. I am biased toward the cream version because you not only insert it in the vagina, but you can also put it on the vulva, urethra, and clitoris, giving these structures the hormones they need for good collagen and blood flow and function.

Systemic hormones: Think your whole body when you hear systemic. Here, topical estrogen (in the form of a patch, gel, or Femring—yes, that last one goes in the vagina, but it is still systemic) is used to treat menopause symptoms and prevent osteoporosis. If you have a uterus you also need a progestin. This can be oral or through an IUD and is NOT topical unless combined with estrogen in a patch to protect your uterine lining from the estrogen (unopposed systemic estrogen has a 5 to 10 percent uterine cancer risk).

Vaginal hormones: This is low-dose vaginal estrogen (in the form of cream, tabs, or a ring) that is used to treat or prevent GSM. It does not treat other menopause symptoms as it is only local in the pelvis. Using vaginal hormones DOES NOT require any type of progestin to protect the uterus.

Can you use both? Yes! Totally allowed! In fact, systemic hormones may not be enough (remember they are still quite low dose, offering way less than you had in your twenties, when you were pregnant, or on birth control) to make their way into pelvic structures to treat GSM. Some experts say 20–50 percent of people on systemic hormones still need a vaginal one to help with GSM.

When women complain to me that estrogen cream is too messy, it definitely makes me smile. Put it in before you go to bed and it is often gone by the morning, or use a slightly smaller dose to get the job done. Also, do you remember how "messy" your vagina was in your twenties? There was so much discharge. That's actually called a healthy vagina. Dry is not good, my ladies.

Besides, we do plenty of things to make our life better. How many creams do women put on their faces? They never think, *Ugh, another cream. I'm not doing it.* They're like, *Oh, this was eighty bucks and it's amazing. I'm going to use it because it's going to help my under-eye circles and fine lines.* Vaginal cream does even better things than that, and it costs way less!

I had a patient I'd cured of bladder cancer come in for a scope to make sure there hadn't been a recurrence. You know what she told me? "What REALLY saved me was vaginal estrogen! My clitoris doesn't hurt anymore, I'm not getting UTIs, when I have sex I am lubricated, and my tissues feel soft." How's that for a blockbuster review? Of course she was relieved to be in remission from bladder cancer, but a life-changing improvement happened when I properly diagnosed her genitourinary syndrome of menopause. She had been to two nurse practitioners and two other physicians with these symptoms and just kept getting put on antibiotics.

Vaginal estrogen now comes in a generic form, so make sure your provider prescribes that. Shop around for the best price by using the GoodRx app and typing in your zip code and medication name. This may seem like a pain, but this is a medication you need to be on for decades (symptoms return when you stop). Saving money in this case means saving A LOT of money. Currently generic vaginal estradiol 0.01 percent cream is thirty dollars at Costco in my town.

There are risks to any medication—even the most basic thing that you can get at the corner drugstore. If Tylenol came on the market now, some experts claim it would never be over the counter because if you take too much of it, it can cause liver failure. In the case of systemic estrogen, the risks include blood clots (lower risk than pregnancy and oral birth control) and vaginal bleeding. As for vaginal estrogen, it is so safe I think it should be over the counter. The risks listed on the package insert are wrong, and the American College of Obstetrics and Gynecology has been petitioning to have this changed for years. Left as is, it scares women and forces them to decide between their doctor's advice and the FDA's. I tell women up front that the package warning is incorrect with regard to the true risks of vaginal estrogen, and that they can trust me on this one, but I am sorry to contradict the FDA. I am sure this doesn't engender trust in your doctor or the FDA, but they aren't changing the labels as of this writing and women need not fear unnecessarily.

My soapbox for vaginal estrogen is that it's like sunscreen and safety belts. Chapstick for the vagina and vulva. Yoni essential oils. I actually think it should be a preventative medicine. Here is your mammogram, colonoscopy, and vaginal estrogen. Consider starting it in your fifties to prevent the atrophy, shrinkage, pain, tearing, dryness, bladder symptoms, and UTIs that happen to 50 to 80 percent of women and only get worse with age. A woman's atrophy in her seventies is often way worse than in her late fifties.

It doesn't matter whether you have menopausal symptoms or not. As your ovaries stop making estrogen, this is what happens to your vagina and vulva. Why have pain and dryness in the first place? Let's keep our organs healthy. It's better to prevent problems now than to try to reverse damage after ten years of low hormones. Britain's health service has realized how much money will be saved by treating women with estrogen up front instead of treating the diseases caused by low estrogen later in life. They are not only supporting women with menopause clinics, they are keeping it very affordable.

People can be so judgy when it comes to HT, but why do they care? Do they want to deal with your osteoporosis, hot flashes, and painful body parts? Do they care that your quality of life and sex life could well decrease due to menopause symptoms? If it seems like hormones are right for you, go talk to your doctor. It's your body; you have to live in it and take care of it responsibly like no one else does.

Sadly, though, even doctors can be judgy about hormones. I just saw a woman in her midfifties whose doctor had stopped her systemic hormones without explanation. She didn't question him because she didn't want to be perceived as difficult or argumentative, so now she was having recurrence of her menopause symptoms (it's no coincidence so many women get a urology referral six to twelve months after stopping hormones when the consequences on the pelvis start kicking in). *WHAT?* I wanted to scream. *It's your body! Go back, understand why, or seek a second opinion.*

If your doctor isn't willing to give you HT, understand why first. Some women can't take systemic HT secondary to history of blood clots, genetics, stroke, liver or heart disease, actively getting treated for breast cancer, or beginning them more than ten years after reaching menopause. In most of these situations, it is still safe to take vaginal estrogen. So if someone told you "you can never take estrogen," it is likely they weren't thinking about low-dose vaginal estrogen and you still may be able to. If those are not the reasons, please go see a different provider instead of ending up in a clinic that wants to charge you large amounts of money for proprietary compounded hormones or put pellets in your body. Most women who have to pay for their hormones stop doing it anyhow—it is just not sustainable. Besides, compounded hormones and pellets are not regulated and can be very high dose with worse side effects, like a clitoris that grew to the size of a small penis and may not ever go back to normal. True story; I have seen this.

Stop Should-ing on Menopause

What about the thought that "menopause is natural" and you shouldn't take anything for it? My response is, if you want to be all-natural, don't have air conditioning. Don't wear shoes. Get rid of your car. You can't have modern conveniences and then tell people they shouldn't have vaginal estrogen.

Besides, if "natural" aging was the norm, everyone should just take off their glasses right now. No one NEEDS glasses—can't you get by with squinting and using a magnifying glass? Dry skin, painful childbirth, dying in childbirth, cancer, and sunburns are also natural, but we don't sit idly by. We prevent and treat. Take agency for your sex life and hormones.

Also remember a natural thing that happens after menopause is a silent 2 percent decrease in bone mass every year leading to epidemic costs, frailty, and death secondary to hip fractures (elderly women have 80 percent of the three hundred thousand hip fractures in America every year). You can't feel that happening, but you can decrease your risk significantly with hormone therapy. So "only take hormones if you feel symptoms" is a myth that you don't have to abide by. See your personal physician for your specific risk/benefit analysis, or check out menopause.org to find a NAMS-certified provider.

I'm not here to argue with the "natural" police. You do you, but don't tell other women what to do based upon a made-up "natural is better" story. Instead, challenge what you consider natural. Maybe you're just saying that because you're scared of hormones, don't want to take medication, or are just trying to figure out what to do.

If a guy came in saying he had brain fog, would any doctor tell him to just live with it? No! No doctor tells a man with low testosterone it is normal and to learn to deal with it. And yes, testosterone "naturally declines" with aging. Are there side effects to taking testosterone? Yes. And there are also risks with living with low testosterone. I think once you look at it that way, you realize how patriarchal it is to tell women what they should or should not do during menopause.

We don't "should" on men like we do women. I have the great privilege of seeing all genders. We don't hold hormones back from trans individuals or cis men, but we do to women—all in the name of "protecting" them. I call bias.

Until I started podcasting and really hearing women's stories from around the world, I had NO idea how hard it is to advocate for sexual and menopause health. Understanding the "why" behind your doctor's reason is not being argumentative or difficult. It is a signal of agency, understanding, and getting on the same page as your provider.

I see women in every decade of their lives and I see what is possible for us. Care for your body and you can have enjoyable sex for your entire life. And while you're at it, stop should-ing over menopause!

You Are Not Broken

N o one is going to give you permission to work on your sex life. Okay, I am. And your future self is.

Maybe your significant other, too.

Damn it. Now you have potentially three people giving you permission. But you only need one person's permission—your OWN. You are worthy of good sex because you exist and you were born in a human body. It is no more complex than that. Stop waiting to "get over" something or to find the magic pill, partner, or toy.

What would your future self tell you about the adventure of discovering your sexuality? Is she satisfied? Is she happy you put in the work? What does she want you to know and try? Your best advisor is your future self.

There is no set formula to a great sex life. You now have all the concepts and ideas you need to get started. Go learn, try, fail, try again, and refine. Sex never ends. It's just like exercise or being healthy.

As you age you must adapt, prioritize, communicate, and continue to come back to the practice. Good sex isn't an accident. It doesn't happen TO YOU, it happens BECAUSE of you. This is a lifelong practice. No one is so good at sex that they can't get better.

As Tony Robbins said, "It's not about the goal. It's about growing to become the person that can accomplish that goal." What matters most is who you become on the journey. What you learn in the process of becoming the woman with the sex life you desire is the goal. This is different than desiring the outcome. The journey is the whole point. That involves self-acceptance, optimizing your health, body confidence work, becoming more accepting of pleasure, having better communication with your partner, being in the moment, and staying present when sexual. Enjoy the ride. Have fun with it.

Of course, you won't have a better sex life just by reading a book—even this book. If it was that easy, everyone would have an amazing sex life. You have to DO! So:

- Go into the bedroom and prioritize your pleasure.
- Accept that your body is normal and worthy the way it is. It doesn't need to look like or be anything other than what it is.
- Cultivate nonperfectionist expectations.
- Don't "should" yourself. Treat your body and thoughts with kindness.
- Tell yourself, *I love myself enough to have a happy sex life.*
- Educate your daughters and sons about sex and the female body.
- Teach another woman what you've learned.
- If you wish you had known all this—that's how everyone feels. Make others feel understood. Bring up the conversation.
- Give others this book if they need it (unless you took notes and don't want to share—in that case, gift them another copy).

- If this book changed your mind about sex, use that information to change the conversation in society.
- If you still need professional help, see a sex therapist and a trusted physician. This is not a sign of failure; it is a sign of you advocating for your needs. Get a second opinion if you need to. I guarantee with the info in this book, you will be so ahead of the game and ready to have an educated conversation with any therapist or provider.

In the end, it all comes down to identity. Shedding the identity given to women by society about how sex is "supposed to be" in heterosexual relationships. Shaking the beliefs that hold you back. Leaving behind the shoulds, lack of education, and lack of empowerment given to us to own our sexuality.

Our society and religions are ever-changing and impermanent. There is no better time to find out the truth about your sexuality for yourself. Like a scientist, don't take anyone else's word for it.

You now know that spontaneous desire isn't necessary for magnificent sex. That desire is created or killed by you. And that your level of desire is enough and not to be compared or judged next to anyone else's. You can purposefully increase desire by being intentional with your thoughts, feelings, and actions.

This is literally ancient wisdom. The Dhammapada, a collection of Buddhist sayings, states, "Hard it is to train the mind, which goes where it likes and does what it wants, but a trained mind brings health and happiness."

Only YOU get to decide what you desire. And there it is again... desire. Whatever you want, you can get. You are already worthy. You are already enough. And

YOU

ARE

NOT

BROKEN

Acknowledgments

So much love and gratitude to:

- My mom, who saw the doctor in me long before I did and showed me what writing a book looks like.
- My brother Hans, who is my rock and closest thing to a mirror in my life.
- My podcast listeners and women who share their "broken" stories, and time and again push me to keep sharing this message and my dharma with the world.
- Dr. Jimmy Turner and Dr. Amy Vertrees for insisting a book needed to happen.
- Dr. Sunny Smith for pushing me toward life coaching and coaching me out of my dabbler and job-y ways.
- Dr. Rachel Rubin, my East Coast sister. Thank you for fact-checking me and all the love and support—let's keep f*ing changing the world!
- Trish Cook for helping me turn my passion into this book.
- Dr. Irwin Goldstein, who told me I was a future leader in this space—and I believed him.
- To that annoying voice in my head—my future self—telling me I needed to start talking and sharing this information with the world. I will follow you anywhere.
- My husband for never thinking I'm "too much."
- My girls—may I show them what is possible.

Resources

I've assembled the "best of the best" information I found on my journey to becoming a sexual medicine expert in case you, like me, want to keep learning and growing your knowledge in this area. And like, why wouldn't you want to do that? The more you know, the better your sex life can be. Woo-hoo!

Organizations

International Society for the Study of Women's Sexual Health
    (ISSWSH)
North American Menopause Society (NAMS)
The American Association of Sexuality Educators, Counselors, and
    Therapists (AASECT)

Coaches for Sex

The Life Coach School
Sonia Wright at soniawrightmd.com
Yours truly on my monthly live podcast recordings (more groups in
    the future as time allows) kellycaspersonmd.com
alexandrastockwell.com
daniellesavory.com

Books

I am a bibliophile and literally have read dozens of books before I decided yes, the world did need my unique voice in this arena. Here are some of my favorites.

Better Sex through Mindfulness: How Women Can Cultivate Desire by Lori Brotto

She Comes First: The Thinking Man's Guide to Pleasuring a Woman by Ian Kerner

Magnificent Sex: Lessons from Extraordinary Lovers by Peggy Kleinplatz and A. Dana Ménard

Becoming Cliterate: Why Orgasm Equality Matters—And How to Get It by Laurie Mintz

Come as You Are: The Surprising New Science that Will Transform Your Sex Life by Emily Nagoski

Mating in Captivity: Unlocking Erotic Intelligence by Esther Perel

Love Worth Making: How to Have Ridiculously Great Sex in a Long-Lasting Relationship by Dr. Stephen Snyder

Women's Anatomy of Arousal: Secret Maps to Buried Treasure by Sheri Winston

Never Split the Difference: Negotiating As If Your Life Depended On It by Chris Voss

The Body is Not an Apology: The Power of Radical Self-Love by Sonya Renee Taylor

Menopause Manifesto: Own Your Health with Facts and Feminism by Dr. Jen Gunter

Estrogen Matters: Why Taking Hormones in Menopause Can Improve Women's Well-Being and Lengthen Their Lives—Without Raising the Risk of Breast Cancer by Avrum Bluming and Carol Tavris

Rekindling Desire by Barry McCarthy and Emily McCarthy

Podcasts

You Are Not Broken by Dr. Kelly Casperson
Life Coach School Podcast by Brooke Castillo
Women's Health by Heather Hirsch

Websites

omgyes.com
meetrosy.com
mojoupgrade.com
dodsonandross.com
Quiv.re

Citations

INTRODUCTION

1 https://cfmedicine.nlm.nih.gov/physicians/biography_35.html
2 https://www.ncsl.org/research/health/state-policies-on-sex-education-in-schools.aspx
3 https://sites.bu.edu/dome/2021/01/24/theres-no-such-thing-as-sex-without-consent/

CHAPTER ONE

4 https://www.prnewswire.com/news-releases/texas-voters-support-abstinence-plus-sex-education-in-schools-a-new-bipartisan-poll-shows-301078365.html
5 https://www.youtube.com/watch?v=JKKRBnpDpBY
6 Witt, Charlotte, and Lisa Shapiro. 2016. "Feminist History of Philosophy." In *The Stanford Encyclopedia of Philosophy* (Spring 2016 ed.), ed. Edward N. Zalta.
7 G. Baht, A. Shastry, "Average Time to Orgasm (TitOr) in Females during Heterosexual Penovaginal Intercourse," *J Sex Med*. 16, Issue 6, Supplement 3, S6, June 01, 2019 DOI: https://doi.org/10.1016/j.jsxm.2019.03.469.

CHAPTER TWO:

8 https://medium.com/radhika-radhakrishnan/what-being-a-sex-positive-feminist-means-to-me-b7cf21fd25ce.
9 Herbenic D, Reece M, Sanders S, Dodge B, Ghassemi A, and Forten-

berry JD, "Prevalence and characteristics of vibrator use by women in the United States: Results from a nationally representative study," *J Sex Med* 2009;6:1857–1866.

10 Barry McCarthy, JMST, https://www.huffpost.com/entry/partner-doesnt-want-sex_n_6518638.

CHAPTER THREE:

11 Michael E. Metz & Barry W. McCarthy (2007) "The 'Good-Enough Sex' model for couple sexual satisfaction," *Sexual and Relationship Therapy*, 22:3, 351–362, DOI: 10.1080/14681990601013492.

CHAPTER FOUR:

12 https://wexnermedical.osu.edu/blog/myths-and-facts-about-hymen

13 Lloyd, J., Crouch, N.S., Minto, C.L., Liao, L.-M. & Creighton, S.M. (2005) "Female genital appearance: 'normality' unfolds," *British Journal of Obstetrics & Gynaecology* 112:643-646.

14 Beale, D., Miles, S., Bramley, S., Muir, G. and Hodsoll, J. (2015), "Nomograms for flaccid/erect penis length and circumference," *BJU Int*, 115: 978-986.

15 https://ohnut.co/

16 Joseph A Kelling, MD, Cameron R Erickson, MD, Jessica Pin, BS, Paul G Pin, MD, "Anatomical Dissection of the Dorsal Nerve of the Clitoris," *Aesthetic Surgery Journal*, Volume 40, Issue 5, May 2020, pages 541–547.

CHAPTER SIX:

17 Parish SJ, Simon JA, Davis SR, Giraldi A, Goldstein I, Goldstein SW, Kim NN, Kingsberg SA, Morgentaler A, Nappi RE, Park K, Stuenkel CA, Traish AM, Vignozzi L, "International Society for the Study of Women's Sexual Health Clinical Practice Guideline for the Use of Systemic Testosterone for Hypoactive Sexual Desire Disorder in Women," *Climacteric*, 2021 Apr 1:1–18.

18 Goldstat R, Briganti E, Tran J, Wolfe R, Davis SR, "Transdermal testosterone therapy improves well-being, mood, and sexual function in premenopausal women," *Menopause*, 2003 Sep–Oct;10(5):390–98. doi: 10.1097/01.GME.0000060256.03945.20. PMID: 14501599.

19 Goldstat. *Menopause*, Sep–Oct 2003;10(5):390–98.

20 Ensieh Fooladi, Robin J. Bell, Fiona Jane, Penelope J. Robin-

son, Jayashri Kulkarni, Susan R. Davis, "Testosterone Improves Antidepressant-Emergent Loss of Libido in Women: Findings from a Randomized, Double-Blind, Placebo-Controlled Trial," *The Journal of Sexual Medicine*, Volume 11, Issue 3, 2014, Pages 831–839.

21 https://www.jsm.jsexmed.org/article/S1743-6095(20)30982-6/fulltext

22 Arnot, Megan and Mace, Ruth, "Sexual frequency is associated with age of natural menopause: results from the Study of Women's Health Across the nation," *R. Soc. Open Sci* https://doi.org/10.1098/rsos.191020.

CHAPTER SEVEN:

23 Marin et al. "Misattribution of musical arousal increases sexual attraction towards opposite-sex faces in females," *PLoS One.* 2017; 12(9).

24 Meston CM, Frohlich PF, "Love at first fright: partner salience moderates roller-coaster-induced excitation transfer," *Archiv Sex Behav*, 2003;32(6), 537–44.

CHAPTER EIGHT:

25 Roy J. Levin (2011), "The human female orgasm: a critical evaluation of its proposed reproductive functions," *Sexual and Relationship Therapy*, 26:4, 301–314, DOI: 10.1080/14681994.2011.649692.

26 Haake P, Krueger TH, Goebel MU, Heberling KM, Hartmann U, Schedlowski M, "Effects of sexual arousal on lymphocyte subset circulation and cytokine production in man," *Neuroimmunomodulation*, 2004;11(5):293-8.

27 Davey Smith G, Frankel S, Yarnell J, "Sex and death: are they related? Findings from the Caerphilly Cohort Study," *BMJ*, 1997 Dec 20–27;315(7123):1641–44.

28 Erdman B. Palmore, PhD, "Predictors of the Longevity Difference: A 25-Year Follow-Up," *The Gerontologist*, Volume 22, Issue 6, December 1982, Pages 513–518.

29 Frederick, D.A., John, H.K.S., Garcia, J.R. et al., "Differences in Orgasm Frequency Among Gay, Lesbian, Bisexual, and Heterosexual Men and Women in a U.S. National Sample," *Arch Sex Behav* 47, 273–288 (2018). https://doi.org/10.1007/s10508-017-0939-z.

30 Willis, M., Jozkowski, K.N., Lo, WJ. et al., "Are Women's Orgasms Hindered by Phallocentric Imperatives?" *Arch Sex Behav* 47, 1565–1576 (2018). https://doi.org/10.1007/s10508-018-1149-z.

31 Lara Eschler (2004), "The physiology of the female orgasm as a prox-

imate mechanism," *Sexualities, Evolution & Gender*, 6:2–3, 171–194, DOI: 10.1080/14616660412331330875.

32 Franco MM, Pena CC, de Freitas LM, Antônio FI, Lara LAS, Ferreira CHJ, "Pelvic Floor Muscle Training Effect in Sexual Function in Post-menopausal Women: A Randomized Controlled Trial," *J Sex Med*, 2021 Jul;18(7):1236-1244.

33 Frederick, D.A., John, H.K.S., Garcia, J.R. et al., "Differences in Orgasm Frequency Among Gay, Lesbian, Bisexual, and Heterosexual Men and Women in a U.S. National Sample," *Arch Sex Behav* 47, 273–288 (2018).

34 Kontula O, Miettinen A, "Determinants of female sexual orgasms," *Socioaffect Neurosci Psychol*. 2016;6:31624. Published 2016 Oct 25. doi:10.3402/snp.v6.31624.

CHAPTER NINE:

35 Nicolas Guéguen (2009), "Mimicry and seduction: An evaluation in a courtship context," *Social Influence*, 4:4, 249–255.

CHAPTER TEN:

36 Dewitte Marieke, PhD, Carvalho Joana, PhD, Corona Giovanni, MD, PhD, Limoncin Erika, PhD, Pascoal Patricia, PhD, Reisman Yacov, MD, PhD, and Štulhofer Aleksandar, PhD, "Sexual Desire Discrepancy: A Position Statement of the European Society for Sexual Medicine, *Sex Med*, 2020 Jun; 8(2): 121–131.

37 *Enduring Desire: Your Guide to Lifelong Intimacy*. Michael E. Metz, Barry W. McCarthy. 2010.

38 Karen E. Sims & Marta Meana, "Why Did Passion Wane? A Qualitative Study of Married Women's Attributions for Declines in Sexual Desire," *Journal of Sex & Marital Therapy*, 36:4 (2010), 360–380, DOI: 10.1080/0092623X.2010.498727.

CHAPTER ELEVEN:

39 Hayes RD, Dennerstein L, Bennett CM, Sidat M, Gurrin LC, Fairley CK, "Risk factors for female sexual dysfunction in the general population: exploring factors associated with low sexual function and sexual distress," *J Sex Med*, 2008 Jul;5(7):1681-93.

40 van Anders, Sari M et al., "The Heteronormativity Theory of Low Sexual Desire in Women Partnered with Men," *Archives of Sexual*

Behavior, 1–25. 23 Aug. 2021, doi:10.1007/s10508-021-02100-x.

41 *Enduring Desire: Your Guide to Lifelong Intimacy*. Michael E. Metz, Barry W. McCarthy. 2010.

42 Heiman, J.R., Long, J.S., Smith, S.N. *et al.*, "Sexual Satisfaction and Relationship Happiness in Midlife and Older Couples in Five Countries," *Arch Sex Behav* 40 (2011), 741–753. https://doi.org/10.1007/s10508-010-9703-3.

CHAPTER THIRTEEN:

43 van Anders, Sari M. et al., "The Heteronormativity Theory of Low Sexual Desire in Women Partnered with Men," *Archives of Sexual Behavior*, 1–25. 23 Aug. 2021, doi:10.1007/s10508-021-02100-x.

44 Kontula O, Miettinen A, "Determinants of female sexual orgasms," *Socioaffect Neurosci Psychol.* 2016;6:31624.

CHAPTER FOURTEEN:

45 Berman L, Berman J, Miles M, Pollets D, Powell JA, "Genital self-image as a component of sexual health: relationship between genital self-image, female sexual function, and quality of life measures," *J Sex Marital Ther*, 2003;29 Suppl 1:11–21. doi: 10.1080/713847124. PMID: 12735086.

46 Woodard TL, Nowak NT, Balon R, Tancer M, Diamond MP, "Brain activation patterns in women with acquired hypoactive sexual desire disorder and women with normal sexual function: a cross-sectional pilot study," *Fertil Steril.* 2013;100(4):1068–1076. doi:10.1016/j.fertnstert.2013.05.041.

47 Rehman US, Rellini AH, and Fallis E, "The importance of sexual self-disclosure to sexual satisfaction and functioning in committed relationships," *J Sex Med*, 2011;8:3108–3115.

CHAPTER FIFTEEN:

48 Goldstein et al., "Hypoactive Sexual Desire Disorder: International Society for the Study of Women's Sexual Health (ISS-WSH) Expert Consensus Panel Review," *Mayo Clin Proc*, January 2017;92(1):114–128.

49 J.L. Shifren, B.U. Monz, P.A. Russo, A. Segreti, C.B. Johannes, *Sexual problems and distress in United States women: prevalence and correlates,* Obstet Gynecol, 112 (5) (2008), 970–978.

50 Maseroli E, Rastrelli G, Di Stasi V, Cipriani S, Scavello I, Todisco T, Gironi V, Castellini G, Ricca V, Sorbi F, Fambrini M, Petraglia F, Maggi M, Vignozzi L, "Physical Activity and Female Sexual Dysfunction: A Lot Helps, But Not Too Much," *J Sex Med*, 2021 Jul;18(7):1217-1229.

51 Johnson, M. D., Galambos, N. L., & Anderson, J. R., "Skip the dishes? Not so fast! Sex and housework revisited," *Journal of Family Psychology, 30*(2) (2016), 203–213.

52 Andrea Salonia, Giuseppe Zanni, et al., "Sexual Dysfunction is Common in Women with Lower Urinary Tract Symptoms and Urinary Incontinence: Results of a Cross-Sectional Study," *European Urology*, Volume 45, Issue 5, 2004, 642–648.

53 Jaspers L, Feys F, Bramer WM, Franco OH, Leusink P, Laan ETM, "Efficacy and Safety of Flibanserin for the Treatment of Hypoactive Sexual Desire Disorder in Women: A Systematic Review and Meta-analysis," *JAMA Intern Med.* 2016;176(4):453–462.

54 Lynn BK, López JD, Miller C, et al., "The Relationship between Marijuana Use Prior to Sex and Sexual Function in Women," *Sex Med*, 2019;7:192–197.

55 Landén M, Eriksson E, Agren H, Fahlén T, "Effect of buspirone on sexual dysfunction in depressed patients treated with selective serotonin reuptake inhibitors," *J Clin Psychopharmacol*, 1999 Jun;19(3):268–71.

56 Fooladi E, Bell RJ, Jane F, Robinson PJ, Kulkarni J, Davis SR, "Testosterone improves antidepressant-emergent loss of libido in women: findings from a randomized, double-blind, placebo-controlled trial, *J Sex Med*, 2014 Mar;11(3):831–39. doi: 10.1111/jsm.12426. Epub 2014 Jan 16. PMID: 24433574.

57 Vowels LM, Vowels MJ, Mark KP, "Uncovering the Most Important Factors for Predicting Sexual Desire Using Explainable Machine Learning, *J Sex Med*, 2021 Jul;18(7):1198–1216.

58 E. Sandra Byers Ph.D. & Larry Heinlein PhD, "Predicting initiations and refusals of sexual activities in married and cohabiting heterosexual couples," *The Journal of Sex Research*, 26:2 (1989), 210–231.

CHAPTER SIXTEEN:

59 Susan E. Trompeter, Ricki Bettencourt, Elizabeth Barrett-Connor, "Sexual Activity and Satisfaction in Healthy Community-dwelling Older Women," *The American Journal of Medicine*, Volume 125, 1, (37–43).

60 https://www.jsm.jsexmed.org/article/S1743-6095(20)30982-6/ fulltext

61 https://www.menopause.org/docs/default-source/2017/nams-2017-hormone-therapy-position-statement.pdf.

62 Kay, Alexander. Alexander, J.L., Kotz, K., Dennerstein, L. et al., "The effects of postmenopausal hormone therapies on female sexual functioning: a review of double-blind, randomized controlled trials." *The Canadian Journal of Human Sexuality*, vol. 13, no. 2, summer 2004, p. 126.

63 Dennerstein L, Lehert P, Burger H, "The relative effects of hormones and relationship factors on sexual function of women through the natural menopausal transition," *Fertil Steril*, 2005 Jul;84(1):174–80. doi: 10.1016/j.fertnstert.2005.01.119. PMID: 16009174.S

64 Comhaire, F., "Hormone replacement therapy and longevity," *Andrologia*, 48 (2016): 65–68. https://doi.org/10.1111/and.12419. Paganini-Hill A, Corrada MM, Kawas CH, "Increased longevity in older users of postmenopausal estrogen therapy: the Leisure World Cohort Study," *Menopause*, 2018;25(11):1256–1261. doi:10.1097/GME.0000000000001227.

65 Col NF, Eckman MH, Karas RH, Pauker SG, Goldberg RJ, Ross EM, Orr RK, Wong JB, "Patient-specific decisions about hormone replacement therapy in postmenopausal women," *JAMA*, 1997 Apr 9;277(14):1140–47. PMID: 9087469.

66 Jiang, Xuezhi MD, PhD1,2; Bossert, Anna DO1; Parthasarathy, K. Nathan MD1; Leaman, Kristine MD1; Minassian, Shahab S. MD1; Schnatz, Peter F. DO1,2,3,4; Woodland, Mark B. MS, MD1,5, "Safety assessment of compounded non-FDA-approved hormonal therapy versus FDA-approved hormonal therapy in treating postmenopausal women," *Menopause*, August 2021, Volume 28, Issue 8, p 867-874 doi: 10.1097/GME.0000000000001782

67 https://www.menopause.org/docs/default-source/2017/nams-2017-hormone-therapy-position-statement.pdf

68 Ferrante, Kimberly L. MD; Wasenda, Erika J. MD; Jung, Carrie E. MD; Adams-Piper, Emily R. MD; Lukacz, Emily S. MD, "Vaginal Estrogen for the Prevention of Recurrent Urinary Tract Infection in Postmenopausal Women: A Randomized Clinical Trial, Female Pelvic Medicine & Reconstructive Surgery," February 2021, Volume 27, Issue 2, p 112-117 doi: 10.1097/SPV.0000000000000749 and https://www.auanet.org/guidelines/guidelines/recurrent-uti

Printed in the USA
CPSIA information can be obtained
at www.ICGtesting.com
LVHW040739070124
768299LV00026B/128

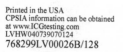

9 781544 524344